Our
Own
Words

Reflections on living with mental distress and extreme states (and living without them)

a collaborative book

inside out & associates australia

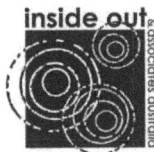

inside out
& associates australia

ISBN: 978-0-646-80664-8

Cover design and typesetting by Mahlie Jewell, Graphics for Good
www.graphicsforgood.com.au

Editing by inside out & associates australia
www.insideoutconversations.com.au

eBook formatting by Michael Hanrahan Publishing
www.mhpublishing.com.au

This book was written to expand perspectives and understandings of a diversity of experiences and does not constitute psychological, medical or any other kind of professional advice. It should not be used as the basis for any decision on the topics it covers. inside out & associates australia and the authors disclaim all responsibility and liability to any person, arising directly or indirectly from any person taking or not taking action based on the information in this book.

The content of each chapter is the sole expression of its author, and those views are not necessarily shared by inside out & associates australia or the other contributors to this book. Certain names and identifying information have been changed to protect privacy.

This book is dedicated to everyone – collectively and individually – who draws on their own experiences of living with distress and extreme states to make the world a better place. In particular, we honour the life and work of Frances Monro, a contributor to this book and to the collective movement, who passed away before publication. We pay our respects to everyone who has lived and worked in ways that enlarge the cultural space to speak about experiences of distress and extreme states in their own words.

Contents

Preface

This project is important to inside out & associates australia. Our approach is based on the premise that better responses to 'mental distress', 'extreme emotional states', 'dangerous gifts', 'alternate realities', 'psychological crisis', 'mental illness', 'spiritual awakening', (or whatever language people choose for themselves), depends on better understanding these experiences, and how people make sense of them. As such, this is not a book that aims to reinforce old stereotypes, limiting perspectives, or clichéd messages. Rather, it aims to share the distinct, creative and unexpected ways that people navigate complex experiences, in a way that readers can relate to and learn from ... and even be surprised and challenged by!

inside out first put the word out about the Collaborative Book Project in early December 2018, circulating a flyer inviting people interested in 'co-authoring a book that will help change the way people think about mental distress/extreme states'. The response, in a very short period of time, was overwhelming. By Christmas over 85 people had contacted us, and in January 2019, 62 people had signed up to co-author this book. Unfortunately, for a range of reasons, 10 people were unable to follow through with their plan to contribute.

There was no selection or culling process. Wanting to contribute to the book project was enough. inside out didn't seek out particular perspectives or particular people to write for the project. People (co-authors) were asked to: "write about an aspect of your lived experience of mental distress/extreme states that you feel holds important learning for yourself and others" with a firm limit of 1500 words.

This fostered a diversity of stories in a book that was not too lengthy to publish and distribute. Editing was kept to a minimum. Co-authors were invited to be as active as they wished to be in shared decisions about the book title and cover, and as co-owners of the book, they will receive an equal share of any funds raised from sales, as well as having the right to promote and sell the book.

After eight months of writing, editing and reviewing, deliberating over possible titles, considering potential cover designs, proof reading and print setting, we had our prototype collaborative book, Our Own Words – Reflections on living with mental distress and extreme states (and living without them), ready to launch on Kickstarter, a crowdfunding platform, through which we hoped to generate the funds to produce and distribute Our Own Words. Thanks to 307 amazing supporters and backers (acknowledged individually at the end of this book) we did it! And here it is. An incredible diversity of stories and poems covering a wide array of perspectives, experiences and reflections. Contents in the book range from the focus on an hour in an author's day, to experiences and reflections over the course of an author's lifetime.

This book is not about people's stories simply as a means to raise 'mental health awareness' or to illustrate the real life experience of mental illnesses, as defined and described by professionals. It is about recognising the legitimacy of lived experience knowledge as central to informing how we think about and respond to mental distress as individuals, families, communities and within systems. The insights that come from navigating these complex human experiences are valuable to all of us regardless of whether we ourselves are struggling or have struggled with distress experiences or not. It's about acknowledging that these experiences are what it is to be human, and their meaning is as diverse as human beings themselves – whether it be a spiritual awakening, a dangerous gift, a life crisis, a trauma response, a psychological emergency, a mental illness, or a super-sensitivity. At the same time these diverse meanings are both uniquely individual, and collectively shared.

We thank each of the authors for their contributions to this project. We are deeply honoured to collaborate with you.

Sandy Watson & Kath Thorburn
inside out & associates australia

Imposter Syndrome
Frances Monro

> *"You gave me hyacinths first a year ago;*
> *They called me the hyacinth girl."*
> *-Yet when we came back, late, from the Hyacinth garden,*
> *Your arms full, and your hair wet, I could not*
> *Speak, and my eyes failed, I was neither*
> *Living nor dead, and I knew nothing,*
> *Looking into the heart of light, the silence.*
> T. S. Eliot. *The Wasteland.*

The woman sat on the train. Let us call her Frances. She sat on the train as it rocked and rattled across town. See brown train tracks and a shiny silver beetle train. The city sparkles in the heat, the river a sluggish brown snake winding among hot streets.

Imagine the woman, Frances, slumped in the seat. Maybe she has a window seat – she likes to look out the window, maybe she gazes out the window at the hot city. Picture her reflected in the glass: square face, messy brown hair pulled back. Narrow mouth. Not a feminine face at all, not a pretty face. A dumpy woman sitting slumped on a train, not worth a second look. Invisible.

Her eyes are her best feature, weak blue eyes, tired blue eyes. A tired woman sitting on a hot train as it rocks slowly down the track. Slowly, endlessly. She is going to see her psychiatrist.

Frances sits withdrawn, staring out the window, silent. Is she really looking at the city? Does she really see it? She couldn't tell you. The endless journey ends and she gets off the train onto the hot platform. Her feet stride over the pavement, sensible shoes pace out the ground: right foot, left foot... Frances walks on automatic pilot, eyes open but thoughts turned inward, expression gives nothing away.

Frances feels sweaty. Her heart races, her thoughts spin. She is going to see her psychiatrist and it fills her with fear. She must explain herself, choose what to reveal, tell her story, try to convey the experience of being Frances. In words.

She always does this. Doctors, dentists, psychiatrists, they fill her with fear, they make her palms sweat and her thoughts race. It has happened so often that she's even aware of it, she's learned to manage it: make it a little ritual.

Leave early, get the early train. There's nothing worse than being late when you're anxious. Stop for coffee on the way. What if the train is late? What if it's cancelled? Frances, you always do this: there's plenty of time!

Stop for coffee on the way. This is her little ritual. Step into the coffee shop, practiced smile for the cashier, order, always the same order. As a transsexual, social interactions are hard for Frances. Have they read her? Will they be hostile? Will they accept her? Do they think she is a man or a woman? Frances, calm down! It's just coffee!

Psychiatrists don't recommend drinking coffee if you're anxious: it's a stimulant, it will just make your anxiety worse. Oh, but it's a little ritual, sitting quietly, sipping, breathing deeply, a chance to relax. Frances needs any chance of relaxation she can get, she's a bundle of nerves, hypervigilant, jumpy. A little social ritual, a smile, a greeting from people you know. The woman has practically no family, few friends, she lives for her work, much of the time her only company the voices or the music in her head. Let her have her coffee: there are worse things than a little caffeine.

Today, however it doesn't work. She's still jumpy and anxious as she leaves the cafe and heads up the street for the tram stop. The ritual has failed. It wasn't a familiar cafe. Maybe the vibe was off? Staff too busy? Coffee not good? Anxiety about losing her purse in her bag? Or maybe it's hormonal? Is she dehydrated? It might be any of these things. God knows Frances is sensitive. She should chill the fuck out but it does no good telling her: believe me, I've tried.

Striding up the street for the tram, the poor girl is on the verge of a panic attack. Sweating, obviously, pulse racing, breathing fast, stomach cramped. But she forges on bravely, pushing herself. God knows she's not a quitter, anything but: she pushes herself too far and then breaks down. Stupid really, stupid, for someone so intelligent.

Dimly she's aware that something is wrong, but she's busy, she'll push through and deal with it later. And there's no reason for her to be so upset! It's irrational! Her doctor is not that scary. She doesn't usually react this badly... this is... madness.

Waiting for the tram. The tram arrives, squeaking and groaning. The doors slide open and she climbs on board.

What is a tram? Picture a green box on steel wheels. Cream wood and glass and leather seats, domed metal roof. Ferryboat feel, an antique, an heirloom deliberately maintained with chugging compressor and squealing wheels. And no air-conditioning.

It's packed. A sea of faces. No seat for the woman on the verge of collapse. No one will make eye contact, no one will look at her, a sea of faces but no smiles, no connection. The sea feels hostile today. The tram puffs and groans its way up the hill, as tired as the woman.

A terrible fear begins to grip Frances and she is suddenly convinced that she doesn't exist. Nobody will look at her because she's not here. At the very best her body might be here (although she feels confused about that) but she's not here, or she's not a human being, or, well she just doesn't exist.

"Get out of my way!" a woman snarls, still not making eye contact. Frances's body moves aside but Frances is gripped by the distressing conviction that she isn't in it. The tram stops and Frances stumbles out to emerge standing in the heat, panting, trembling with the belief that she's not here at all.

Let's break there for a moment, shall we? There are things we should discuss. But wait, you ask, who are you? Who's telling this story? Good question my friend! Call me Critic, and I shall call you Observer.

And what do you observe? The tram chugging away up the street. Frances, her body at least, standing at the tram stop in front of the supermarket. And Frances, well, she's gone, or at least she's convinced herself in a panic that she doesn't exist: it can be a most uncomfortable feeling.

But Frances is tough and she'll be back. She's better able to cope with dissociation than most people, indeed she usually enjoys it: laying down her sense of self and becoming one with the music, or being the process of creation, or holding herself in suspension so she can experience the world directly with her senses.

She has stepped back now to let me talk through her here, she's a little bit worried that I might not go away afterwards! Maybe she's right when she says she doesn't exist? She could make a decent case for it. And who are we to judge? I certainly don't exist and neither do you.

And can we be too hard on Frances if she has dipped out on us under the strain? She is not a mature personality or a strong one: you can bet she didn't use that name when she was a little boy growing up.

Then why do I call her she, why not he? Get fucked. You can fuck right off.

Look, I am Frances' inner critic. I am the voice of rationality, of truth, of objectivity, of authority and decency and civilisation! Yes, I was against this whole transgender thing from the beginning. It made no sense. It was irrational. It was crazy. It was untrue. It was shameful. I could not reconcile it.

But you know, I've changed my mind. Let her be a girl if she's so set on it, if it is necessary. Who does it harm? She has... talents that only unfold this way. It sparks joy. It gives her space to breathe. Space to live. Room to exist. If you will only give her space... leave the girl be: she has done her time.

I will say this though: you're in a pretty bad way when your inner critic feels compelled to defend you.

So, the woman stands in front of the supermarket. The edge has come off her panic, she's coming down. She still feels numb, unreal, shaky, she's still not quite convinced that she's really there, but she can manage. It's not far to her psychiatrist now, an easy walk.

But... she was supposed to pick up dinner at the supermarket. There is nothing she wants less than to go in there, to face people and choices in this shaky worn out state, still half convinced of her own nonexistence. But... after the doctor, she will go straight home, and there's nothing to eat. By that time, she will be tired and hungry, and she will need food.

So, with a deep sigh she plunges in. I told you she was tough.

Supermarket. Do you need me to describe it? White box, fluorescent lights, grey lino, the beep of cash registers. They make you walk through the produce aisle first. Frances pushes a trolley, drifting through the store, half present, can't quite connect with herself or with the world.

She stops by the vine ripened tomatoes, selects some and raises them up to her face, sniffing deeply. The scent floods her nostrils: tangy and viney, and so, so, real. She can feel them in her hands, she can smell them so vividly it's like taste.

These tomatoes are realer than I am... then her mouth quirks and she begins to laugh.

Fran Monro is an experienced mental health peer support worker and trainer from Melbourne. Fran delivers training to new peer workers around best practice in peer support, and training to non-peers from a lived experience perspective. She role-models recovery on a daily basis. She is passionate about dancing and jazz music. Fran believes seeking joy and living each day to the fullest. She is known for breaking into song with no excuse.

Meds to Mindfulness
John Shearer

My story begins in 1982 when I was driving an old 1418 Mercedes Benz truck on the Hume Highway near Kilmore in Victoria. Suddenly, out of thick fog, the back of a stationary truck appeared. I didn't even have time to think and yanked on the steering wheel in a hopeless effort to avoid a crash. That's the last thing I remember until I regained consciousness in Kilmore hospital. I found out later that I died in that accident and was revived at the scene. There was no white light or any sort of after death experience, just blackness. Coming back however, was an unforgettable experience which I still cannot find words for. The solid steel bonnet of my rig rolled up, smashed through the windscreen, and killed my dog instantly. The bonnet actually finished where we had been sitting.

I have no doubt that my guardian angel was with me that day and somehow I was thrown clear of the carnage. I had a conviction in me that I was somehow saved for a reason, so I started a quest. I studied history, religions and cultures. Little did I know that my battle was only just beginning. I had multiple physical injuries but that was nothing compared to the psychological impact on my life. One minute, I was living a normal family oriented happy life and the next, it was taken away from me. It wasn't long after the accident that I started suffering from stress and anxiety. My mind was like a drunken monkey, very busy and all over the place! I turned to drugs in an effort to ease the pain and slow down my mind.

Later that year, I had my first vision and chased after it. I was unable to catch that vision and spent time in a mental health unit at the local hospital. I was told that I had experienced psychosis. Depression followed and I was labeled 'manic depressive.' Medication was given in an effort to level out my moods. I had more visions in 1984, 1987 and 1992. Each time was a different story with the same result, hospitalisation and heavily medicated. The depression in between the highs was more severe each time. All sorts of drugs were used with little effect. At one point, electric shock treatment was used, but it seemed that there was no hope. I was told by medical authorities that I would never be cured, never work again and would have to take medication for the rest of my life.

By 1997, I was rock bottom. I was ashamed that I had mental 'illness' and refused to talk about it or get help from outside the 'system'. It was my dark secret. Later that year, I had another vision. It was a Monday and I was at Central Station in Sydney waiting for a train back to my home town. As I started walking along a very long platform, I was suddenly aware that I was making eye contact with all the males. One by one, they glanced at me, looked me in the eye, acknowledged me with a nod or made some sort of gesture. When I got to the end of the platform, my head was in a bit of a spin. There was plenty of time until the train was scheduled to depart, so I decided to walk back on the other side. I was amazed at what happened next. The same thing occurred, but this time it was all the females!

"Oh no!" I cried out to myself. "Not again!" I thought I was having a fifth 'manic' episode but this time I thought quietly "If this is you God, you can come to me this time. I'm not going to chase after this anymore!" I decided to put it behind me and let it go.

On Friday that same week, I answered a knock on the door and got a very pleasant surprise. It was an old friend who I had not seen since before my accident. It turned out that he had moved to Sydney to become a professional punter. He visited owners and trainers to gather information about their horses. He was very successful and built a house, got married and started a family. Eventually however, gambling got the better of him, and he lost everything. He went on to tell me his story, how he had hit rock bottom and was then saved by the power of the Holy Spirit.

"Do you believe?" my friend asked. I then told him that I only believed in the Dark-side and shared an experience that I had ten years before. It was five o'clock on a very cold morning in May. I had woken from a very bad dream. I was terrified. I left the house, dressed only in shorts and singlet, and started to run. I didn't feel the cold or my bare feet, all I felt was fear. I ran over five kilometres and ended up on the bank of the Murrumbidgee River at dawn. It was my favourite place and for a moment, I felt peaceful. Suddenly, a powerful message became apparent in my mind. "Kill yourself or your youngest child will die!" I screamed at the top of my voice, "NO! F**K YOU! GO AWAY!" I then collapsed onto my knees and broke down in tears. I picked out a gum tree and seriously considered suicide. A tiny voice in the back of my mind said, "There's a reason, you'll get through this." Later that day, I ended up back in hospital.

My friend prayed for me and suggested that I go to a meeting at a private house on Sunday. He explained how it was a Spiritual prompt that made him visit, and a friend was starting a new home church. He then continued his travels and I haven't seen or heard of him since. I am certain that he was indeed, sent by God. It is interesting that the date was 10th October which was to become World Mental Health Day! Two days later, I went to the house on the other side of town. It turned out to be a praise and worship type meeting with music, singing and prayers. A visiting 'elder' asked me if I wanted to give my life to Jesus and be baptised. I said, "Sure! I'm on the road to nowhere anyhow!" He went to the boot of his car and pulled out a portable baptismal tank which was set up in the back yard. I was then baptised by full immersion.

As I came up out of the water, I was praying in tongues. I had never even heard of tongues before that day and have been praying that way ever since. I love the tribal emotion that I feel and the fact that it is prayer from the heart and not the mind. It wasn't like an overnight miracle, but my life slowly began to change. In some ways, it was like waking up from a nightmare and turning on the light. My 'blinkers' came off and I could see things clearly. I was able to stop smoking and go off medication. My daily walk with the Divine had begun and I never fail to feel connected. Most importantly – no more depression! I finally had the black dog securely on a leash.

The incident at the Sydney Railway Station had taught me that we are all connected with each other. My relationship with God/Universe has taught me that we are all connected with Spirit. There are no coincidences in life. When you pray and want something bad enough, things will happen. You will meet the right people, at the right time. I now understand why the Bible is called the Living Word! As I read the Word, God spoke to me. There were heaps of 'ah-ha' moments too! They are moments when your Spirit lines up with Divine Spirit, a kind of 'knowing.' There was one moment in particular that was extremely powerful, much more than any other, similar to the dark epiphany I had in 1987, but this one was from the Light! The message was, "Help the mentally ill!" I remember looking up to the heavens and saying "Whoa! but Lord, I am one of them!" It seemed so ridiculous at the time, but it was to become my passionate purpose. There is no way I could even remotely envision that I would end up with over a million 'likers' of my two Facebook pages. One called

Mindfulness Mentor and the other called Spiritual Warrior.

I value my 'dark' years now because I overcame many fears and learned heaps of life lessons. I now know the truth about what happened to me, it is easy to be wise looking back. In 1982, '84, '87 and '92, I experienced what is now known as Spiritual Crisis or Emergency. I had no way of knowing what was really going on until my old friend shared his story. It was that story that led to my Spiritual Emergence in 1997. I got my life back and have never looked back, except to see how far I've come.

I now know that bipolar 'disorder' is a gift. It's not a gift that you would wish on anyone, that's for sure! But when you wake up to what's really going on, it is life changing. I have had times of 'mania' since 1997: these are simply times when I am totally inspired. I require no medication because I am in control of my mind rather than my mind controlling me. Today, thanks to a well-developed mindful practice, I live with both peace of mind and clarity of mind. Never lose hope my friends, there was a time when hope was all that kept me alive.

John Shearer is an Australian mindfulness master, psychotherapist, spiritual mentor and founder of mindfullyMAD.org (mindfully Making A Difference). He is grateful for his fifteen 'dark' years because it helped him become who he is today. He gained much wisdom and learned heaps of life lessons. John is passionate about his purpose which is helping a world in crisis to awaken. His signature saying is: Be Mindful... Pause... Connect!

A few mad love letters.
Flick Grey et al

Dear suicidal parts,

Thank you for all the ingenious ways you have kept us alive. So often, the mere thought of you has been comforting. You've held hope – a way out – when life felt too overwhelming, when life *was* too overwhelming, painful beyond words.

With mad love and respect,
Flick *et al*

****

Dear suicidal parts (again),

Thank you for offering deep insight into human suffering and creative survival.

We're sorry that we've tended to take you far too literally. You are wise, but your language is cryptic. We're starting to understand that when you whisper in our ears, you are not seeking to *end* life but to *redirect* life – you call for a fuller, richer life.

To be honest, it's a bit embarrassing that you've needed to teach us this lesson several times over now. Sometimes, we turn to simplistic solutions to very complex life problems, especially when we get scared. The mysteries of life are just too big for our human-sized brain. Please try to remember that while you are lateral-thinking, we can be a bit literal-thinking.

When, sometime in the future, you speak with us again, we'll try our hardest to listen deeply to your sweet whisperings, to listen *underneath the surface,* to the depth of your truth. We'll try our hardest to remember that your spiritual and philosophical yearnings are not what they seem, superficially, that your truth is deep and lateral, not superficial and literal.

We're sorry that we've let them call you names, belittle you, medicate you into silence, as if you made no sense. We can see how disrespectful and counter-productive that has been. If we collectively knew how to listen to your wisdom, life would be greatly enriched.

What do you think of the idea of "suicide listening" instead of "suicide prevention" (or "suicide listening as suicide prevention")? Would you be willing to help us understand your mysteries?

When you next come to visit, hopefully we can hold each other more closely and listen deeply to understand your wisdom. Please don't misunderstand, this isn't a call to hold each other close with handcuffs and restraints – they really hurt our spirit, not to mention our wrist and already-dodgy knee. And the medications just made us sleepy. Unsurprisingly, our soul – and our will to live – didn't flourish in captivity. Here's hoping we can find ways to hold each other, with humility and space and deep listening.

With mad love and respect,
Flick *et al*

****

Dear little part who stopped eating,

Thank you for giving us that delicious and intoxicating sense of omnipotence, when we felt so desperately powerless – you were our lightness and closest friend in that expanse of darkness.

Thank you for embodying unspeakable complexities – the intricate and intimate relationships between our body and our boundaries, community and family, what nourishes and what is toxic. You expressed wisdom we had no words for, wisdom that (had we found words) had no space for expression. Some things are forbidden to speak of and you held a silent protest.

We're sorry we let them call you names, like 'anorexia'. It wasn't a lack of appetite. We lacked words. We lacked permission to express ourselves fully, especially the pent-up rage about things that happened to us in childhood. You did such a fine job of expressing the enormity of things we couldn't (yet).

We hope you're not terribly offended if we say that we hope not to need your close companionship again. If we do meet again, we salute your wisdom and will try our very best to listen respectfully. But, for the record, we *really* like ice cream, and apple crumble and kale (but not all together!). We like any food, really, that has been made with love. Actually, we don't like caraway seeds all that much (just saying).

With mad love and respect,
Flick *et al*

****

Dear little part who thought that playing on the train tracks (or climbing on scaffolding) was a better alternative to dealing with life,

You're very clever and brave and adventurous, dear one, but mama says it's time to come inside. We've got your favourite food, loads of picture books, the best sparkly stickers, a trampoline in the living room (for real!) and maybe we could even build a tree-house together, if you'd like?

We know that life can be *really, really, really* hard sometimes. We promise that we'll do our very best to listen to you and take your concerns seriously (and playfully). But we won't allow you to take us all on any more dangerous adventures (we can go on lots of un-dangerous adventures).

You're not in trouble, dear one, it's just that sometimes little people need grown-ups and sometimes grown-ups say "no". Lots of adults are stupid and mean but not *all* adults are stupid and mean.

Do you remember that kind train driver who stopped the train, poked her head out of the driver's carriage and asked if we were okay, before helping us up off the tracks and into her carriage, apologising for not having any chocolate? She was lovely, wasn't she (even if she did say we weren't allowed to take *any* photos, not even of all those amazing dials and levers)?

And do you remember the kind police officer who showed us the tiny ladybird perched on a rock he'd picked up off the train tracks? He was patient and could find that little bit of magic in the chaos.

And do you remember that kind mental health worker in the emergency department who showed us where the treats were stored and then found us the most comfortable chair in the whole ED to sleep in? And do you remember our friend who stayed with us for 17 hours in the ED, even though no one found a comfy chair for her?

And do you remember our friends who went looking for us after we ran away, patiently carrying our big stuffed toy around various parks, and then teaching emergency services how to speak with us?

And do you remember our friend flying all the way from interstate to visit us in hospital?

And do you remember our friend who watered our plants each time we went back into hospital? Not even one plant died!

And do you remember our friend who home-delivered that big box of frozen meals? That felt like a big box of love.

And do you remember that kind nurse whose face lit up when we were re-admitted (again) into hospital? It's okay to miss her – she was really kind.

There have been so many really, truly kind people along the way, even if there have also been many, really, truly unkind and stupid people too. We know you're allergic to incompetence and are so sorry we can't always protect you from it. And, yes, dear one, we agree the system is silly and mean. Please know that there are lots of us trying to change things to be less silly and mean.

With mad love and respect,
Flick *et al*

****

Dear little part who knows that adults cannot be trusted,

Thank you for being the keeper of family secrets – such a heavy burden for one so young. Thank you for protecting us from people who might harm us (more).

Please know that we will listen to *anything* you want to tell us. We hope that, if you come to trust us – if we earn your trust – you'll let us share the responsibility for figuring out which adults can be trusted, and when, and with what, and all those tricky questions.

If you ever feel like telling us about the things that make you happy, maybe together we could figure out how to do *every single one* of them, somehow? Some of them might need to be in our imagination, or we could draw pictures, or make up silly songs? Or maybe some of our creative friends might help us?

With mad love and respect,
Flick *et al*

Flick Grey has multiple parts and passions. With university qualifications in linguistics and social and political sciences, she works as a manager in a peer-run family violence service, freelance consultant and Open Dialogue practitioner. She's particularly passionate about engaging with – and learning from – madness and complexity (and her cat). www.flickgrey.com

Sleeping Giants and Volcanic Scars
Rosie Williams

How to Self Destruct

Chapter 1 -
Allow a slip of the tongue now and then when nobody's looking,
snatch the truth back up and bury it in your pocket
to tumble crumpled into a collection of inky snowflakes in the wash.
Find them again and feel bitter that no one saw their truth.

Cut your heart into breadcrumbs,
spread out for wild animals and *left-over* the earth,
part of you hoping someone will follow.
Try not to care when they scatter it to the birds.

Hide behind braids of flowers in the garden back,
listen with breath baited for hurried footsteps and searching hands -
a solo game of Marco Polo.
Miss a beautiful afternoon
whispering *"I'm here"*
choosing to be lost and losing moments.
Maybe one day you'll find yourself instead.

Hush your heartbeat like a monk's.
Imagine eating monkshood and monkeyhead mushrooms
until it's quiet for good.

Cross the interstate line that separates dreamtime from the world,
curse the violence of longing for a different life.
Hang a vacant sign over the nape of your neck
smacking against your collarbones with every hungry step walked
searching for a better place to lie down.
Make *'I hate myself'* your mantra.

Trace the fossil scar splitting your lip and try to recall the pain
step back from the open mouth of bird hands offering an embrace.
Scan them for sly-fingered fluttering
aching to press hard against your ribcage to check
you're eating.
Use your stone heart to kill them both dead.

Observe the distance between both halves of yourself
chart the separation from others as a million degrees,
then grieve until cool to freezing point.
Break the fourth wall a thousand times and find
no one listening.
Narrate misery to your own company and
fall in love with it.

Chapter 2 -
Feel tears burning a wick behind each eyelid and
refuse to detonate.
Leave the heavy shape of grenades waiting
quiet and unfulfilled.

Say you relate to the Matchstick Girl;
snow tipped fingers outstretched with questions of price -

disguise your naked need beneath frostbite.
Haggle and give out until you rob yourself of a sale.

Let smiles slip through the holes in your soul and
tie bootlaces together so it's easier to trip
and fall into bear traps.
Beg every passing soldier to unclap their jaws.
When no one comes to the rescue,
chew through the gristle and bone until your *sole* is severed loose.
Ruminate on your marrow for years,
while the teeth rust at your feet.
Watch them grin at the world far longer than the wound heals.

Hide scars like stolen heirlooms
curses marking the flesh every transgression.
Carry them like trophies of worthlessness
a mask of righteous martyrdom.

Chapter 3 -
Be too transparently broken to fall in love with.
Despise those that fall in love with your brokenness.
Watch them add sweetener to their words and let it ignite chagrin.
Mix cold water to their burning oils of passion -
decide it's their lies making the air explode.

Pour disquiet over your cereal every morning
bubbling fat and thick with viscous sadness.
When friends and relatives lean too close,
add them to the dark cauldron
as spell ingredients.
Fail to notice that you've hexed yourself.

Light candlewicks on your fingernails
suggesting a meal together in an expensive restaurant.
Use them to cast the curtains into inferno
Molotov cocktails instead of Bordeaux.

Chapter 4 -
Hollow out soil and climb into the grave
persuade anyone who asks that you're comfortable
that it's quiet here
that you're just resting with your arms crossed.
Forget to resurrect yourself.

Sew stones in your pockets instead of skipping them over the lake.
Eat yellow paint, hope for happiness
and cultivate harm –
a bowerbird collecting charms that look like talismans.
Camouflaged monkeypaws and pale rabbits' toes
clasping *hopeless* white-knuckled to the chest,
a secret tattoo.

Paint yourself blue and play guitar with your head bent.
Scare crows into flight until they darken the sky and obliterate the moon,
drown in the starry night of loneliness
open a room of solitude and lock yourself safe.
Tell yourself you'll let down your ladder hair later -
neglect to look out the window for the arrival of a prince.

Chapter 5 -
Weave every perceived rejection into an overcoat
wear it as chainmail and save for a better cloak to transform your life.
Swear like a trooper it's protecting you from bullets and stabs in the back
– tell yourself the heavy ache and bruises are worth the shoulder chips.

Starve your body until the cage of your heart stands to attention like
soldiers refusing to wave a white flag and
lay down their guns.
There's a murmur in the ranks –
abnormal QT waves fluttering in the wind.
Sparks spots your eyes like grim stars on the horizon.
Traumatise your mind so much, your body becomes alien –
Strangelove Syndrome from the brain-stem down.

Ignore the scar tissue in your throat from broken nails of regret
let every unsaid word rake your oesophagus.
Rehearse a script of *I'm unloved* and echo it -
fail to practise other lines.
Remain an understudy in the wings of your life,
Say it's fine, you're not a star but a dying dwarf giant
who'd rather act a supporting part if it helps.

6 -
Romanticise your mushroom rot and decaying wood -
hold up the picture of your sickness like Dorian Gray,
a portrait of immortality and escape.
Paint your eyes with cataracts to blind yourself
spores of living death are too ugly to bother with.

Sigh at your life as Narcissus did, and see how long you can go
until your last breath.
Turns out you should have cut gills into your wrists.

7 -
Conjure enemies from shadows that the sun already bleached.
Dance a tapestry of fear in a fairy ring and
step into it when the moon is low.
Spirit yourself into nothingness
a ghost with a banshee scream as soft as the hoot of an owl;
boo-book, boo-book.
Leave a changeling person in your place,
hoping someone will notice the melting ice and peer into its face.

Plant weeds in manicured gardens as an excuse to poison the ground.
Blame the world for letting those seeds grow in the first place.
Pace in circles to water them lovingly,
tend and knead until their limbs bear fruit.
Watch the fall and fermenting waste.

8 -
Dig for pips, and repeat.

Vortex

Your tongue hits your teeth like a drum
in time with your heart,
in time with mine.
Your words trip fast like fists

beating out of your skull
our hurt as plain as headstones
that we stake deep between the ribs of our earth.

We are tiny satellites
spinning, hidden in this sky.
Broadcasting pain in the vast dark
unfolding our truth in a battlecry that
rips us red and open.
Supernova stars exploding blood
eons and light years apart that will echo and echo.
We will be picked up and felt
for generations down.

I hold space for you and you for me.
We see each other and say
we are enough and we always will be.
I hear you and I love you
the shame and pain you carry was never yours.
Let it be swallowed down through black holes
back to those it belongs to.

We are quasars in a vortex -
our power is immense, beautiful, bright
in this moment we are whole and powerful.
We fall and others have fallen before us
their pieces orbit the skies and guide our healing.
Eyes raised to the heavens see sparks of light
and wonder they're seeing scars of life already gone -
relics of survivors and pain honoured and learned from.

We hear stories and it moves us to our core
I love you and I hold space
I hold space
you are whole and
you are beautiful.

The Locked Wards

Statistics written in skin
naked and sick,
lips hung with words but
hollow of expression.
There is no softening the medicine
trickling into bone.
Dream lucid or speak insane,
mad tones lost to effortless hands
guiding your skeleton to a locked room.

Bound in white
breathing in the scent of stars and faded galaxies
gauze and Betadine and
decaying souls, light already gone.
The florid notes of hope
linger in doorways
ground shut on the back stairs
a two-at-a-time descent.

Pills trespass fairy weights on her tongue
a cloying sweetness rich and thick that is darkness embodied.
Blue sheets billow out their sails and go nowhere -

they moor their anchors in melancholy and the heavy despondency
of the yellow pills and barcodes – drop her eyelids and
shuffle her feet along the ocean floor like a shell-less crab, searching for a
home.

In the night these seeds germinate and bear fruit
What strange leaves she grows.
She loves the flowers and learns
to stay her hands from plucking at the roots -
the nightshades and shadows of her heart
unfold like childhood monsters and imaginings.
Exposed and transformed in twilit morning,
stark bones of shark skeletons turned into lantern cages.
Rest candles in their hungry doors and close them like the
heavy locks of the ward.
She finds her way out,
suitcase zipped and reminiscent of the scars in her mind, on her skin;
survival inscriptions of life and here,
statistics of battles won.

Immersion

Goose-fleshed skin, bathed under fairy lights in bright reds and gold
as warm and whole as you don't feel.
Trembling fingers undoing the clasp of your straps
knotted treble clef of your hair trailing down to the
curved base notes of a spine and hips
too prominent and shook with cold and nerves.
Rising over the crescendo flood and hovering above yourself in the
sweet night air of this pool, you loose your hands into your hair and send
it down – a tsunami of blue.

Pearls dot your skin – fear tattoos
raised quavers in staccato bursts, in time with your tread -
full stops and ellipses of dread… breves of cold unreal.
You hold your semi-breath twice too long,
shame ebbs and wanes its waves.
You draw your lungs in, and let your shirt unravel.

Soft light plays its rays and mallet hands across your ribcage with the
heavier weight
of so many pairs of eyes, and a gasp or two.
They peel your scales back to fish bones, your floundering pulse exposed
with their question mark hooks.
Your heart buoys to the top of its thrumming mast
a deep heave along the strings and vocal chords to your cello chambers;
you manage breath, and unfurl a flag of letting go.

Tiptoe to the water edge;
cool exhilarating blue.
First step into the depths, and you allow your weight
to fall.

You join these bodies in their beautiful
this dance, with a rhythm at once communal and all your own,
until there is a heat building slowly within.
This body deserves its own lovesong, and
there is oblivion, there is a moment of feeling
and being
wholly and
only united
as you.

Rosie (Ruby) Williams is a provisional psychologist, peer support worker, mental health researcher, lived-experience speaker and lecturer. Rosie manages and survives severe-enduring anorexia nervosa, perceptual disturbance/psychosis, different traumatic experiences, self-harm, suicide, and psychiatric restraint and confinement. Rosie believes sharing stories deepens understanding of oneself, encourages self-exploration, growth, and transcendence. She believes in the power of compassion in care as means of transformative justice and healing. Rosie finds healing in poetry, and hopes others find solidarity in her words.

Illness, wilderness, liberation
Matt Ball

What they called illness

As a 21-year-old I had been running, running for many years from practical and more ethereal vulnerabilities. The frantic path, mapped out for me by experiences in my life, shuddered to a halt when I ended up in a psychiatric unit. In the months and years prior, I had become increasingly distressed by the experiences in my mind, beginning around the age of 13, hearing voices and fearing that I was being consumed by an entity. The less definable, but no less challenging chaotic states of mind stayed around throughout my teens until the chaos became overly dominant.

Hearing voices and seeing images, fearful and chaotic, I was diagnosed and labelled and admitted to a brand-new psychiatric unit on the site of an old asylum. As a child, I had joined in the stereotyping of the old asylum, and the people within the confines of that 'mad house'; then I became one of the mad people! Despite seeing myself as somehow different to the other people in the hospital, it turned out that my somewhat inevitable destination had arrived. From pseudo sanity, I arrived in a place I belonged.

Hospital admission led to a diagnosis of depression and psychosis. Diagnosis led to being medicated. Diagnosed and distressed, I accepted the labels and drugs as a legitimate narrative. Discharged – hearing voices and suicidal – I accepted that the 'treatment' by psychiatry was of value as part of the chemical imbalance (mental illness) theory, that had been described to me.

Four further admissions followed and I spend most of 18 months in hospital. Coerced into poly pharmacy including anti-depressants, mood stabilisers, antipsychotics and benzodiazepines. Electroconvulsive therapy (ECT) was administered voluntarily – unless of course I decided to leave or refuse ECT – and then I was to be detained: I was labelled with the diagnosis of 'schizophrenic illness'.

During the barbaric psychiatric 'intervention' of being placed in a padded cell, I was to experience what would later become a theme for me in making meaning and new understanding. The theme that followed me from the early years to today is the spirit and power of human connection. When secluded in a cell, one member of staff put his head in each hour and said 'I am just wanting you to know I am here. I have not forgotten you. Please don't tell anyone I have come to see you, I am not supposed to communicate with you while you are in here'. He was not allowed to communicate with me, but he couldn't resist the compassionate intention to connect as a human being.

Accepting the medicalisation of my distress, I soon began repeating a story to professionals that provided a face saving (for me) rationale for my madness: this story provided a rationale for diagnosis and treatment for the psychiatrists. However, this simple story belied the secrets of shameful, confusing and unspeakable realities.

Implausible as it seems now, I also accepted psychiatrists telling me that their drugs worked, but also that I was responsible for my wellness. However, when not following the prescription of drugs, admission and ECT (because it didn't 'work'), one doctor told me "you will never get better because of your behaviour and unwillingness to change".

The double bind was something I felt, experienced and knew. I remember asking in ward round "what is the difference between your drugs and street drugs?" My medical notes show that the interpretation of this question was that I was being 'rebellious'. Reflecting now, I was speaking to a 'knowing' of the non-sense that was being offered as a medical approach.

Wilderness years

The wilderness years began as I emerged from a foggy drug (medication) haze. I was living in a housing community with others who were said to be mad, the beautiful support and connection created by three incredible 'staff' invited un-madness to emerge in me. Over time I engaged in voluntary work with older persons, and people with physical and intellectual support needs.

Going on to train in counselling and psychotherapy, exploring Buddhism and reconnecting with my spirit, was liberating. Attending university for the first time, to become a mental health nurse, saw me explore whether the wilderness: its somewhat barren and benign landscape based on the original story of diagnosis and treatment, was actually a reality I still accepted.

The wilderness became an inquiry into either acceptance of diagnosis or rejection of mental illness, and was both a wonderful and strange time. Gratitude and happiness emerged from no longer being in the mental health system, and a sense of discovery (mostly about my own mind) really felt good. This was embodied when running a marathon in 2005. I trained and ran alone using Vipassana meditation. It was an intention to observe, as consciously as possible, all that was present in the process and experience of running hundreds of miles, and a reflective commitment to be as conscious as I could of my mind in my life. It was liberating to observe my mind and spirit in a challenging situation: what I began to observe was the un-madness of being mad when not being labelled as mad. What does this mean? Well if you ever run a marathon you will hear many of your own 'voices' as the struggle of being at the limit of bodily safety emerges. But I was not labelled anymore. I was learning that the labels and ideology of psychiatry were simplistic, unfounded, false and based in its power and authority over truth. I observed the same energy and intensity of narrative when isolated and training for marathons as I had as a 'patient', only this time I felt powerful enough to observe and be aware of the experience without expressing this externally.

For the most part in the wilderness I observed great peace. Though more empowered, discontent and discomfort did begin to emerge when I was working in psychiatric settings. These settings exposed me to an awareness of experiences that may have happened to me, as I witnessed them happening to others.

Speaking out in those settings was clearly difficult for everyone. I found that as I did speak out, I again observed my mind, this time with more understanding and choice, as to the knowledge I accepted. My mind, not mad but a place of complexity in the context and environment of challenges.

Professionally, I began to find permission to work and be in relationship in a way that was more about connection and humanity, and less about accepting things that were illogical and didn't make sense (professional certainty). My supervisors and friends, especially Mary D and Denise B, spent many hours supporting me to find my power, providing a window to new meanings. This led me to develop some understanding of my own and other people's madness, through human to human connection and bringing together the threads of people's lives, distress and humane encounters, towards healing.

The garden of liberation

The current iteration of understanding my madness began one October day in 2011! During my first shift in an Emergency Department in South Australia, I witnessed a person in distress being shackled to a bed. I had never been in a mental health setting where this had happened before. I was shocked and overwhelmed. I could not believe what I was seeing. This crude abuse of a person in distress brought a crashing end to the fading sense of the wilderness years.

A new awakening was upon me. My connection to self and to others in mental distress was clear, and my responsibility apparent. This period of my life would deliver intense learnings, as I was confronted with trying to understand the experience I had faced in the mental health system and the narrative of my life, but with a twist: now I was educated, empowered and no longer had dust in my eyes.

Although I had always known that the approach of others to my distress was mis-attuned, I was now clear that the narratives others had told on my behalf, and the silences I had maintained due to shame, guilt, culture, were no longer a truth for me.

The truth of my past regrettable actions, the actions of others and the swarm of stories that had informed my life (many of which were the stories of others) were clear. The labelling and representation of my distress, by psychiatry and the mental health system – as a biological disorder – and worse the double bind of illness and blame, now held some clarity for their non-sense and ideological control and power.

In exploring my own journey and finding meaning in the emergence of 'psychosis' as meaningful in allowing my emergence from distress, I inevitably found a responsibility to seek to facilitate the same humane opportunity with others. Discovering the experiences that shaped my life, understanding the chaotic internal and external reality, has been invaluable. Seeking to speak this truth in the spirit of openness and curiosity, and in the witnessing of the narrative of another person, has been a new journey. Deeply listening to the narrative of others has been liberating personally, and has offered new meaning professionally.

The learnings from my own journey have become meaningful: I, as a mutual learner, moving towards connection with others, and moving away from flaccid acceptance of oppressive psychiatry. I am walking alongside people in the wilderness of emergence. The diagnostic constructs of understandable distress can otherwise be understood by a person, in the context of their own life, as a potentially meaningful reality. Being alongside a person navigating the path towards their own garden of liberation, has become the privilege of my life.

Matt is a Mental Health Nurse Practitioner and psychotherapist. Matt developed the explanatory framework – 'Dissociachotic' – a concept that explains and provides understanding of how 'psychotic' realities are better understood through a dissociative lens; both emerging and evaporating within the human to human relationship. Matt is Founder and Co-Director of the Humane clinic (www.humaneclinic.com.au). His work is informed by his lived experience of madness and un madness – both in his personal and professional journey.

Turning my life around for the better – one step at a time
Jenny Smith

I grew up in a house with a Dad who was unwell. We did not realise back in the 80s the behaviours he was displaying were due to mental illness. We found out the hard way in 1992, after a couple of psychotic episodes, when we realised there was something really wrong with Dad. We did not know where to get help, no one explained anything to us, we were pretty much on our own. No one seemed to talk about it back then like we do now.

In the late 90`s my sister became unwell. Some of the help she got was good, while other help was not so good. It felt like we were going around in circles for her to get better. In my own case I was diagnosed with depression and anxiety. I got better quickly due to being on the right medication.

Nevertheless, my own life journey has been very difficult. I was bullied in primary and high school: I never had many friends, I found school work too difficult so I failed – no help was ever offered so I did not bother too much about doing homework or handing in assignments. As for work, I was always in and out of jobs, courses and government programs that were meant to help me find work or gain skills to get a job, but then when I applied no one would ever give me a chance to prove myself. I got rejection after rejection. I even tried going to university as a mature age student to start a teaching degree, but I failed at that too, so I made the decision to leave after one year. I did not realise all those years ago that the answer was staring me right in the face, how I could make a contribution to society and lead a fulfilling life.

Mum and my sister were already mental health educators. Mum had been doing it for many years speaking to various groups of people about mental illness from a carer's perspective, then my sister joined as a consumer educator, and has been talking to various groups about her own experience.

I was undecided about whether or not to take the plunge and become an educator myself. I knew I had a story to tell and it was my story: I grew up in a home that had a strong history of mental illness. I was always interested in education and making a difference, but the thing that was holding me back was the greatest fear of all: public speaking – I hated it! Any time in the past that I had to get up and present something, I did everything to avoid the situation.

I applied for the Mental Health Educators program and my application was successful. When I spoke to the facilitator beforehand, she was so excited that three members of the one family were going to be sharing their stories as educators. Two days of training were next on the agenda, and they were very intense. We were trained in how to write the story of our lived experience of mental illness, in public speaking and presentation skills.

After training, I spent time writing notes, and plenty of them. I typed up my speech – I spent nearly an entire day working on it. Editing was the next step and I did end up changing a few bits and pieces and refining it to incorporate the important stuff people would want to know. The next step was one more meeting with the facilitator to practice my speech and refine it again after she made a few suggestions. To my surprise I was told a job was available speaking to volunteers about my experience. I was not expecting that at all so soon after training, and I did hesitate at first, but accepted it in the end. Strike while the iron is hot, I thought.

I met the volunteer coordinator who seemed nice, and was keen to have me on board as a speaker. I was excited by the opportunity but also a bit nervous as it was my first time.

The day before my presentation I was speaking to one of the staff. The first question I was asked was "are you nervous?'" I said, "a bit" but did not really let on that I was feeling very nervous about my first presentation. We had a bit of a chat and she told me everything would be fine after the phone call. I practiced my speech, I put my notes in a folder and did not look at them till the next day. The night before I was feeling a bit anxious about it all because it was my first time. I had my fingers crossed it would go really well.

Presentation day finally arrived. I was feeling very nervous. I tried not to think about it when I was going to the venue, I tried just to go with the flow of it all. I arrived at the office and met up with the staff in the education and training division of the organisation. By now I was not feeling good at all – the butterflies really started to kick in. One of the staff volunteered to come into the training room with me, as she wanted to be the one to give me the thumbs up from the back of the room. The support I got from the staff was fantastic. While I was waiting, I had a chance to look over my speech one more time before I went outside to join the group of volunteers for morning tea – I did not have much too eat, there was not a lot time and I was talking to the facilitator about what was going to happen when we got into the room.

This is the moment I wasn't looking forward to. I took one deep breath and walked into the training room. I was familiar with the room as I had done training there before. I quickly walked up to my seat to join the other speaker who was also presenting. We were formally introduced to the group and I was asked to speak first – the spotlight was on me. I could feel my heart racing, so I took a deep breath and started to give my speech one line at a time, one paragraph at a time. I finished the first page, I encouraged myself to keep going, I was feeling more confident as I went on. I got a shock after I noticed that I was halfway through my speech. I took another deep breath and told myself "keep going you can do this". I was on the home stretch now, only one more page to go, I`m getting close to the end. I could not believe it – I finished my first speech. I took a deep breath and was so relieved that I had done it, I felt fantastic. After a sip of water, I had my question and answer session. None of the questions were problematic. I tried to answer them as best as I could so that the group would have a better understanding of mental illness and how it affects families. I breathed a sigh of relief when my section of the presentation was over. I felt really good and pleased my part had gone so well.

At the end the of the session the facilitator thanked us for sharing our stories with the group, and we had a round of applause from everyone. The facilitator spoke to me afterwards and said that I did a great job, she was happy to have me back in the future. We then left the room and returned to the office. The staff were really happy that my presentation went well, they gave me a lot of praise, and I was feeling really good about myself at that stage. I deserved a pat on the back after what I had achieved!

I was on cloud nine and really happy to have conquered my fears. I got a phone call from the program coordinator a few days after my speech. She wanted to touch base with me and enquire as to how I got on with my presentation, since it was my first time and she was not there on the day.

Doing something like this proved to me I can do just about anything. Subsequently, I have been featured in their newsletter as a success story and my lived experience story was included in their annual report in 2016. This experience really gave me the confidence to try other things. I am now a volunteer within a few mental health programs, I sit on a number of committees and have just become a board director for a non-profit organisation.

I am a person with lived experience of mental illness, I am a volunteer within the mental health sector, my roles currently include youth mentor, peer support, mental health educator, and advocate I am a member of a number of committees and have recently been appointed as a board director for a non-profit organisation. In my spare time I like to surf the internet, keep in touch with friends & supporters via social media.

Walking through Madness
Nicky Bright

One of the fondest childhood memories I have is the soothing sound of
my father's voice reading one of my favourite story books which was the
'Adventures of the Wishing Chair', by Enid Blyton. I can recall that feeling
of security and how I would most often try to delay or postpone going
to sleep because of the occasional nightmares that would greet me once
my eyes were closed. Reading this book to my youngest child many years
later is where I re-discover and understand how I likely identified with
the stories within this impressionable fairy tale. Through reflection upon
these experiences I can see how I would have identified with the magic,
the wishing, the curiosity, and the bonds between parents and siblings.
I can also identify common themes in the interpretations of my dreams
whereby I would be left speechless in times of distress, and confused and
helpless in my attempts to escape unpleasant environments. I see now
why I would evidently yearn for the sense of security I found in those
precious moments.

Venturing into adulthood, I continued to sit by my family's side as
they narrated their own stories and searched for their own meaning
making, purpose and hope. Over the years I began to recognise that
certain stories were drawn upon during times of great frustration, stress,
sadness, tragedy or loss. I listened to many explorations of alternate
realities, spaces, and places, and felt incredibly fascinated by these
stories. Simultaneously, I was somewhat perplexed as to how my family
had discovered these explanations, and had access to experiences that
I couldn't see myself, and that weren't being relayed from a novel. My
curiosity remained and at times I would hear things I could identify with,

such as experiences we had shared, though they were being told from a different worldview in that moment. I did not seem to have complete access to the magical and intriguing visions and places they spoke of such as the 'snakes under the bed', 'diamonds dripping from our faces', 'deceased family members nearby', or the 'seven angels' of protection. Biblical verses were recited word for word without a bible on hand, and almost prophetic insights into our futures or those of others we knew, were foreseen. Some of those insights came to fruition.

For many years most of my frustrations, angst and fears were surfaced by the apparent contradictions between what I was hearing, feeling and understanding of these events, against how these were being defined, understood and explained by others. Those explanations seemed disappointing, non-translatable, and quite distant from our lives.

In my younger years, it appeared to be those responses, or other interpretations, that disconnected us from extended family and the general community, and kept us at a distance. I grew more distressed and fearful of where my family would be taken after sharing these expressions and why it was necessary for our connection to be monitored, limited or isolated. For many years, I accepted my family's interpretations of these events, yet at the same time grew increasingly frustrated by the authority of others whom seemed to be contributing to the new narratives inscribed into our life story. Their narratives and explanations seemed worlds apart from ours and as such inaccessible to our understanding. An 'illness' narrative did not seem to fit, nor did it when comparing our circumstances to other patients within a hospital or even, in comparison to the pain or discomfort of physical illness.

I had noticed from a young age that other people with illnesses were not segregated, gazed upon with suspicion, spoken to abruptly or kept in locked wards – which often have bars across accessible exits. Families, friends and communities would usually appear to respond to illness with kindness, flowers, empathy and connection; whereas our experiences seemed to separate us, kept us hidden or rejected, criticised, frowned upon, silenced or at the worst, spoken of as a demonic curse. The world seemed to insist that I was living and walking through madness. Madness that was a curse which should be excised, removed, suppressed or, as the more authoritative voices would insist, required chemical or physical interventions, and in its most extreme forms, legislative control. The difficulty in accepting this was that I was made to believe these experiences were not things that one should express. These stories should not be told, nor heard. Although I may not be able to understand the necessity of harmful, forceful and coercive interventions, it would be in our best interests to comply. We were told time and again that these experiences were illness, and that to avoid further distress, isolation and disbelief we should accept the narratives and treatments that they recommended.

The most treacherous chapters throughout my life were the moments spent by my loved one's side where all too often I felt like a bystander. I did not see illness. I heard stories, and shared much interest and curiosity. I would desperately try to remain attentive before a disconnect was imposed upon us – physically or chemically induced. This pattern would teach me that submission and compliance were the only ways to alleviate any forms of distress. There were no alternatives for three of my loved ones, and no room for alternate understandings. Fear was inscribed in those transactions, those moments – times when the making of these judgements on our lives, our identities, and our stories was deemed a necessity. These interpretations were being made via a different lens to the one through which we were looking.

There was a pivotal point in my life where I grew to feel so weary, frustrated and deeply despaired by these narratives that I became physically unwell. I had adopted various 'imaginary tools' and attempted to use them in hope of replicating that sense of safety I knew in my younger years. It got to a point where I seemed to run out of 'tools' and felt I had to wear the defeat. The pain of loss, separation, sadness, confusion, and fear had become all-consuming and I couldn't seem to find that sense of safety. I began to submit to the idea that perhaps we were ill, broken, too much, too little, unacceptable and most certainly crazy. I surrendered and met with a psychologist who sat with me for a while through this undoing. She listened to me deeply and validated my experiences with attentiveness, empathy and curiosity. We worked together for a while until she suggested an alternative pathway that could contribute to the transformation I had longed for and convinced myself I needed. There was a difference in this instance, because she supported me in resisting the transcript a psychiatrist had drafted in a half hour meeting, and briefing, of my family history. In fact, she resisted it as strongly as I did because she understood that it would hold no purpose for me in moving forward with my life; and that had it been published, I may have succumbed to the same reaction I had strived so desperately to free myself from. This opportunity for agency and choice felt unusual to me. I was given a choice – to hear that the psychiatrist judgements were based upon my family's medical history – or I could hear the hope someone else was offering, having walked with me for a while, and heard my story.

I chose hope, and the opportunity to explore new meaning. This is where I discovered my purpose.

My name is Nicky Bright, I am a wife, a mother, a sibling, a friend and a Social Work student. My Lived Experience as a carer and consumer ignites an emancipatory vision and commitment to listening deeply to the voices of those who are most often marginalised, oppressed or excluded in our communities. I aspire to facilitate people's opportunities to explore the meaning, purpose and hope found within their own unique stories.

Out of the Ashes
Trys Reddick

I was diagnosed with Anxiety, Agoraphobia, OCD and Social Phobia aged 12. I moved to a bustling city from a more laid back small town at 12 and, after having a couple months off school with a dislocated kneecap, I fell behind. My confidence was shot to pieces and I was easy prey for bullies. I didn't transition well from primary to secondary school and, coupled with the secondary school resembling Alcatraz, I started having anxiety about going at all. After a few short months, the Department of Education accepted, rather easily, that I wasn't going, and classified me as a school refuser. It felt like a huge win at the time. Not every 12-year-old gets told they don't have to go to school, but it taught me to stay at home and so I sleepwalked into Agoraphobia.

I tried a program called a Youth Training Scheme (YTS) on completion of my GCSE's (I'm from the UK), but after four weeks I had another anxiety attack, and quit. A pattern that would last another 15 years was developing to become a stronghold in my head. I went to see my general practitioner (GP) who was amazing. He diagnosed me with Agoraphobia and gave me the option of medication but said, "ultimately you will still need to face the anxiety". On reflection, I declined the medication. I was very fortunate in having an awesome GP who understood mental illness in the early 90's at a time when a lot of GP's and the wider community would often have been very hostile towards it. He instead allowed me to attend an appointment with him every week where he'd listen to me vent and laugh at me (in a nice way of course).

I tried to get out and do things in the 10 years between leaving school and beginning my recovery, but most things I tried were very short lived. I got bored very easily or would feel so anxious I'd quit, often going over things in my head so much the night before that I would talk myself out of doing stuff. For some reason, I found myself particularly drawn to the creative arts especially the theatre, radio and TV. I remember volunteering one day for a local community TV station and ended up working on a live show that finished around 9pm. I was so anxious at the thought of getting home on my own; I had to ask the receptionist if she'd walk with me to the bus stop. Pretty embarrassing for an 18-year-old.

We used to have a fish and chip van that delivered to our suburb on Friday nights and he'd park outside my neighbours' house. I was so crippled with anxiety at that time that I literally couldn't go out to get some chips. Instead we got him to come to the house. I'd open the door slightly, get the chips and give him the money. That was how bad it got.

My first step in recovery came in 1994 when, as a volunteer for a local theatre, I managed to persuade some heroes of mine, comedy writers Galton and Simpson, to come and do a show at the theatre. One of the tools I used in my battle – as suggested by my GP – was to watch comedy shows and I had a considerable collection. Galton and Simpson were writers I admired as they wrote many comedy shows including Hancock's Half Hour and Steptoe and Son. They had retired by that stage but came out of retirement to do a special show for the theatre. It was an evening I'll never forget. I also asked comedy writer Barry Cryer to come to the theatre with his one man show and although that never happened, I did get a phone call from him one Saturday morning. It's always a great day for your self-esteem when your idol calls you up. That got me into a hobby of collecting autographs and I started writing letter after letter to my heroes. It did wonders for my self-esteem to get letters from the likes of Michael Caine, Terry Scott and Edward Woodward. By the time I finished I had a collection of over 150 signed photos and 80 letters, most of them handwritten.

The next big milestone in my recovery was going to see my grandparents in Western Australia. I had grown up with my Mum telling me what a beautiful country Australia is and so I was looking forward to going there for a couple of months. My Nan at that time had Dementia and my Grandad had asked us to help him with her. By the time we got there my Nan was bed ridden, and then while we were there my Grandad had a stroke. Even though we were in an awesome country, it was quite a hard time. We had a visit from the Health Department. They said once we went back to the UK, my grandparents could no longer stay in the unit on their own and would have to go into a home. We had to organise their transition into an aged care facility and get rid of the contents of their unit. During that time, I started attending church and gave my life to Jesus. Even surrounded by the stresses of caring for someone with Dementia, there was a peace about that area I had never felt before. I felt such a strong pull to that suburb and felt that I would one day move there permanently.

On becoming a Christian, I started reading a lot of books, both faith-based and secular books on personal development. They had similar themes and most secular books I read even had quotes from the Bible to illustrate their point. Ideas such as what we dwell on become our tomorrow (as a man thinks, so he is), that the battles are in our own heads and the power of forgiveness. Some of the best authors I found in my search included Adelaide-based writer/illustrator and personal development guru, Andrew Matthews, and the Pastor from Abundant

Life Ministries, Paul Scanlon. I devoured their books and it propelled me in a five year journey of recovery.

One of the main things I took from this period is that anxiety is there to keep us safe from dangers but that our minds often make mistakes by linking perceived dangers with the fight or flight chemical, often leading to phobias and avoidant behaviour. One of the battles I had was with a fear of crowds. Back then, I lived in the UK where crowds can be a nightmare if you're not a fighter. At Christmas Eve, everyone is jostling for position and you can end up being pushed around if you don't fight for your space. My head told me to stay home where there are no crowds and I'll be safe, but I resisted. I believed that my brain had made an error and that crowds were really nothing to be scared of. And so, I set about to prove it. I applied for a job as a Crowd Safety Marshall at a rugby ground. And what's more, I got the job. I remember my first shift, my brain in overdrive, my legs buckling under the strain, sweating and about to collapse in a heap but I made it out alive. I went back to the next shift and the next and after 18 months and a Championship win for the team, I was healed of the phobia.

Just over five years after coming to Australia, I was given the opportunity to return to Australia on a student visa with the aim of staying on permanently after two years. I studied for a Diploma in Community Services which I loved and fell into Job Network, supporting people back into employment. I decided to put down roots and started building a house. I asked the construction company to recommend a suburb as I didn't know the area very well. One condition was that it had to be near a train station as I don't drive. He recommended a suburb south of the river that was undergoing a lot of construction work at the time and had a newly opened train station. It was only when I moved into the new home and paid my first lot of rates that I realised I was living in the same LGA as my grandparents.

I now have my own business running Mental Health First Aid courses for individuals and service providers. I have been doing this for four years now and love that I get to use my own experiences to help and support other people. I can safely say I have been through storms, through tragedies and through hurt and pain. I have lost seven people to suicide but one thing I do know is there is hope. We just need to walk through the storm, reach out and know that when we come out the other end, we will be stronger and taller because of it.

Trys was diagnosed with Depression, Anxiety, OCD, Agoraphobia and Social Phobia aged 12 and left school a year later. This began 10 years of incapacitating mental illness. Only when visiting relatives overseas, motivated to emigrate to Australia, did he start the recovery process, arriving on a student visa nine years later. Trys has worked in Community Services, Rockingham/Kwinana and facilitated mental health awareness training. He runs his own mental health training business and co-founded the Kwinana Alliance against Depression.

The High
Lucy Commisso

The high never lasts,
Definitely not forever.

It's marvellous, makes you warm and fuzzy.
It excites you, makes you feel confident and supported.

Makes you disbelieve;
'how could *I* have been in any other state than this?'

You fall asleep happy, smiling;
You don't want the day to end.

You begin to dream,

They are pleasant;
until they are not.

Time. Space.

You wake and it is like yesterday couldn't have been as rosy.
'How could *I* have ever been that confident, happy, assured?'

But I've been here before—it is nothing new.
And just like the day before;
Tomorrow's something new.

There are two things I know for sure, I've always been a creative and I've always used creativity as a tool for understanding and evolving. Even on the grey days, I'm learning to appreciate my mental health, it builds up my strength and expands my empathy and love.

Feeling my way thru in safe spaces
Amanda Waegeli

My birth was a breech birth, my body was born before my head, so from the beginning, I always saw things a little differently to others. I was the first born, the oldest and only girl born to my parents. I love my parents, and know they did the best they could with the resources they had to raise me. I am so grateful my parents gave me the gift of life. I was reluctant to leave my first home, according to my mother I was a month overdue! I felt comfortable in my mother's womb, the nourishing environment protected me from the real world, it was a safe place to be.

Having a physically and emotionally safe environment in which to grow and learn, to navigate life's ups and downs, and to just be, are enormously important to my mental health. Finding places where I can just be who I really am, to be loved, accepted and appreciated for who I am, are especially important when I'm struggling emotionally. I believe enthusiastically that my mental health challenges were not about what was *wrong* with me but more about what was *happening* to me in emotionally and physically unsafe environments.

I know we are all different, but I have always been a sensitive person, who wears my heart on my sleeve, and I feels things deeply; a person who is more comfortable in emotion than in intellect. When I was younger, I was told, repeatedly, "you're too sensitive" … "you're too deep" … "stop crying" … "don't look so sad" … "you need to harden your heart". The take away message I heard was – don't let your feelings out, keep them inside.

Learning my way in the world as a sensitive, intuitive and empathic person, I soon realised I also felt other people's feelings, sometimes to my own detriment. I was acutely aware of other people's feelings, sometimes even more than they were. When I tried to talk about feelings, even other people's feelings, nobody wanted to hear about them. I was told, "don't talk about that" and "that's none of your business". The message I heard when I was young was that no one wants to *talk* about their feelings.

As a creative person, I learnt early that writing poems and songs, creating art and craft pieces, singing and performing in theatre productions was something I enjoyed. It was also a safer way for me to express and release my feelings and thoughts about the world that I lived in. My experience was that fellow artists, performers and musicians, were *my kind of people:* often sensitive, authentic, and willing to express themselves, feelings and all.

Neither of my parents were religious, and as a child, I was curious and felt drawn to Christianity. Perhaps naively, I thought that 'Church' appeared from the outside to be a safe place inhabited by kind, caring people who weren't afraid to talk about pain suffering and feelings. This part of my journey is a chapter in itself, and my spiritual journey is ongoing. I have, however, developed and deepened my own personal connection to God and consider that spirituality, (that is the quality of being concerned with the human spirit or soul as opposed to material or physical things), aligns well with my values, and often helps me to find hope over fear.

I have personally experienced many traumatic and distressing experiences throughout my life, that have produced, in me, extreme states of emotional distress. My first remembering of such an instance was when at the age of eight. I came home from school and my dad was gone, he had left us to start a new life with another woman. I experienced childhood physical abandonment, which led me to first thinking that the world is not a safe place. Disenfranchised grief, and ambiguous loss, left a gash in my growing heart that bled uncontrollably, and felt like the rip was irreparable.

The emotional abandonment which followed was silent, unspoken, almost invisible, and because of this my young mind struggled to make sense of it. All I knew was that something was *not quite right*. I no longer felt emotionally safe, and was not provided with an emotionally safe environment necessary for my healthy childhood development. I coped as best as I could with what I had as a child, by trying to hide who I really was, hide what I really felt. Somehow, I managed to discard the emotional part of me, in order to be accepted and not rejected, and survive in this crazy mixed up world.

Moving forward 25 years, I found myself yet again emotionally abandoned, shut out, this time within a physically violent marriage. That emotional part of me that I had had to hide as a child started screaming at me to listen, literally, and all of my feelings came crashing out like a tsunami. Overwhelmed, I entered the mental health system. Friends, family and doctors confirmed my worst fear, that I was in fact flawed, and that there was something seriously *wrong* with me.

But it was going to be ok, because they, the expert professionals, had a label for me: several actually, and treatments, like medication and ECT, and a safe place called hospital where I could go and stay! Desperate, I surrendered and gave my power away. However, despite ten years receiving the best mental health care and treatment available to treat my mental illnesses, I felt worse: I was numb, and convinced that this world was definitely NOT a safe place to be.

Having my emotional distress pathologized, without taking into consideration the environment I was in, and labelling me with a mental illness has been more distressing, disempowering and disconnecting, leading me to be exposed to even more physical and emotional abandonment in my life. It took away my identity, my voice, my rights, my opportunity to have healthy nourishing relationships with those I love so deeply.

One thing my experiences have taught me to realise is something I already learnt from a young age: that is that most people fear emotions, especially emotional distress, their own and other peoples. In most cases I now understand this to be more about their inability to handle emotions, rather than a fault in me. The art of simply listening and not trying to fix, or do anything, is almost too simple, but obviously way too difficult for the vast majority of people.

When I entered psychiatry – I didn't know then, what I know now – and that is that it just wasn't going to work for me, as a sensitive, caring loving person, who feels my emotions strongly. The environment of a psychiatric hospital for me was cold, toxic, stifling, alien, and oppressive.

The good news however, that I didn't learn from psychiatry but learnt from my peers, is that the medical model is not the only way. I now know there are alternatives and more humanistic ways to find the support you need, in safe environments, from people who will listen, validate, encourage and support you, while you share your experiences and rewrite your own story, reclaiming your own life. This news was enlightening for me, enabling me to begin my personal recovery journey out of psychiatry.

Through finding and being a part of creating safe spaces, I am learning how to maintain my own mental health, outside of the mental health system. Ten years out of the system, as a sensitive, intuitive and empathic person, I feel freer to feel and express my emotions safely. I am open to other suggestions but have learnt not to give my power away in the process of staying mentally healthy.

Nowadays, I prefer to first trust, nurture and nourish the expert within, the part of me that knew all along the value of feeling my feelings, in safe spaces, to help me on my journey. I also draw on and support humanistic approaches to mental distress like: The Hearing Voices Approach, Narrative Therapy, Trauma Informed Care and Practices, Compassion Focused Therapy, Intentional Peer Support, Peer Supported Open Dialogue, and The Power Threat Meaning Framework.

My concerns today have grown out of my deep listening to others, and feeling my own and others' pain. I have a strong sense of social justice, which has directed me to work in areas where I use my lived experiences of overcoming the effects of trauma and adversity, by sharing my lived experience in speaking out publicly, advocating and educating. I do my bit in the consumer movement to help advocate for improvements and better equity for my peers. I work with others to create and support the development of safe spaces, like peer support groups, so people can express their feelings and talk honestly about tough life experiences and move forward. I am inspired knowing I am not alone, and that there are many of us now working to make a difference and make this world a better and safer place to feel and to be.

Amanda is a lived experience trainer and consultant who has worked privately for the last five years. She uses her lived experience of mental health recovery to influence change and improvements in mental health systems for users. In Western Australia she founded Recovery Rocks Community for peers in 2012. She currently lives in rural Qld, and values people and relationships, she enjoys spending time at the beach, playing music and writing.

Of Hope and Pictures
Athena Field

It's early morning and I'm traveling on a train. I can smell the all familiar dread, its potency rising up ready to ruin my day. I'm surrounded by strangers and the smell of coffee and toast. Someone is clipping their toe-nails. This feeling, a very dangerous feeling that is settling in my mind, cankering in the pit of my stomach, is consuming me. I want to disappear and go somewhere that is quiet and dark. I am being devoured. The gluttony of my own ambiguous thoughts provokes that darkness. So dark and so horrid, I am starting to be afraid. It's eating at me from the inside out. The black dog has appeared and I can't handle the obscurity that it is pulling me into its world, the eternal abyss of self-hate and catastrophe. The strangers on the train are oblivious to the narrative that is unfolding before them. I decide that the only way to stop the darkness is to join it. I have this constant feeling of being trapped and not being able to do anything to stop it. The fear and hopelessness eat away at me whilst the silent tears ravage my face and the collapse of my life is all I know and recognise. All anxiety and depression want me to know about how fucked everything is.

I want death.

I'm now lying on a squeaky bed. I can feel the metal bars across my back on the worn-out thin mattress and I can smell the crispness of potent detergent in the sheets. I am being rolled along a corridor, the squeaky wheels singing in unison. All I can see is the dirty ceiling and the lights flashing as I go past. I see people dash from door to door; their blue, white and pink uniforms flash before me. I hear inaudible laughter and screams bellowing from another room. Somewhere, one of the fluorescent lights needs its bulb changed as all I can hear is buzzing, buzzing, and then fading, fading. I remember hearing a siren, I remember the dirty white walls. Someone called out my name. I'm in a hospital. In the psych ward to be exact.

So, began the beginning of a diagnosis and treatment for my mental illness – triggered post-natally, childhood trauma that had never been addressed, and a stressful career that was filled with overwhelming responsibilities, bungled incompetence, tormenting grapevine gossip and vicarious trauma.

Reflecting back on my life, my mental illness symptoms began during adolescence. There were some unspoken traumas of historical abuse that was buried in a foreign land I was never born in but trespassed sometimes through my father's memories and rage towards me. The usual communication problems at home often emanated from a generational gap in translation. A working-class Greek family trying to make ends meet, living in suburbia, brainwashed by cultural governance and socially acceptable ideologies.

I hated the conventional drivel, and wore my Doc Marten boots in church under my long skirt, raising my middle-finger to the mundane. I did well in school, had an enthusiastic eclectic group of friends, and a little sister who kept me amused by her precarious adventures. I was surrounded and inspired by enterprise, although with restrictions from the 'parentals', I never complained, well not always. The good Greek daughter who was hardly ever deluded or dissuaded from normality and acumen. By my mid 20s I paid off my parents' mortgage, bought my dad a car and I entered what would become a successful and awarded career in community services. Eventually I met a wonderful man, and my independence thrived. We did the usual stuff – got married, bought a house, travelled, partied, and progressed our careers. The next step in our journey was to start our family.

And so, began the evolution of my depression. Infertility being the catalyst. Eight years of failed assisted conception treatments, smothered with a handful of diseases such as endometriosis, and other leeching 'iosises' squatting residence in my body. Miscarriage and false pregnancies, weeks spent in bed weeping from grief and absolute failures. I endured and carried on however, raised by my family with vigour and pertinacity, and faith as my secret weapon. The miracle finally transpired on an inconsequential night, and my son eventually entered our lives. I named him after a dove, its meaning – hope.

I looked at my wee child, took a deep breath, thanked God for blessing me and then it hit me like an unpredictable tsunami. What now? Was I supposed to have inherited or be instilled with the skills of Master Parent just because I wanted a baby so fucking much? I was the lucky one and should I now be happy and grateful with the blessing and shoulder the medal for all Parents after Infertility? The overwhelming responsibility and insensible thoughts of perfection devoured my daily existence. I neglected my humanity, buried common sense and engrossed myself with reasons to die. The black dog yelled at me that I didn't deserve joy. That I didn't earn the right to be his mother. It tricked me to believe that I was useless, and that this world was too precious for someone as irrelevant as me. That day on the train, a stranger called an ambulance. My torment was not too conspicuous to the normal decorum of a passenger travelling on a train.

The time I spent in the psychiatric hospital was both profound and challenging. I experienced the overwhelming effects of guilt and surrender. I was embarrassed, confused and exhausted. Yet the treatment and support provided by the clinicians, my family and friends would have a resonating vibration that led to my recovery and the acceptance that it was okay for me to not be okay. The treatment took several attempts to produce a manageable quality of life and wellbeing that consisted of medication, psychotherapy and mindfulness strategies. I would no longer be haunted by the nightmares of a tragic existence, but that of a woman who had a purposeful and meaningful story, and a lived experience to inspire others with hope and recovery who struggle with infertility, and mental illness. Although the black dog likes to visit these days sporadically, its bark isn't as relentless as it used to be. Overall, the final stages of sustaining my recovery had led to a resolution and connectedness to my son. The black dog surrendered to the true love that flooded my whole being.

I practice mindfulness.

I observe the blue texta in my son's little hand. The table itself is already covered in green, orange and red scribblings. I secretly smile that the crayons are water-based and can easily clean off the table once today's art class concludes and nap time begins. Maybe I'll finish my cup of coffee then. He notices me looking at him. Asks me to draw him a picture. I pick up the orange crayon and draw a flower, then the yellow for the sun, the black for a house and the green for three special people who live in the house. His eyes never leave the crayon as it delineates so carefully on the paper. His stare transfixed to the colourful pictures that now fill the blank white page. He tells me he loves me, and that I'm the best mum in the world. He surrenders his arms, and wraps them tightly around me, kisses me on the cheek. He passionately states that I'm his best friend. He curls his tiny body in my lap and falls asleep to the sound of my voice singing. I pray that he dreams of gardens and pretty little butterflies.

You are loved.

It's early morning and I'm traveling on a train. I notice my bum has gone fat. Sitting on this hard surface on this train seat is more comfortable with a cushiony toosh I suppose. Looking out the dirty windows, leaving the tree covered hills behind me. I'm going somewhere. I can't remember as it's not important. The brown fallen leaves rustle and the frosty chill of Autumn weather hugs me. It's nice sitting here, wearing the scarf I crocheted during an art therapy class. It's so quiet. A seat to myself to sprawl on. The carriage is empty – I pick my nose, finger the Tradie undies out of my crack, daydream about my next beach holiday and sipping wine by a serene landscape. No interruptions apart from an abrupt wake up of the train guard's inaudible announcement. It's a nice feeling, this booming silence. This interval from the darkness.

I am resilient.

I'm a woman, a wife, a mother, a sister, a daughter, a mental health peer support worker, an artist and a friend. I also live with depression and anxiety, and my life is more brilliant by this diagnosis. I am passionate about mental health, writing, crochet and showing people that it is okay to not be okay.

I within.
Edward Walter

I cannot remember how it started exactly. My life had not been easy beforehand but afterwards it was incommensurably more difficult. My dreams had become my reality or should l say my nightmares. Of what my hope consisted l couldn't say. It was hidden behind the events which affected how I saw my existence. I had a vague idea of becoming a well-known guitarist in a rock band. After that, when the chemical scalpel had made its incision, l turned to the classical guitar. My teacher, Graham, told me l could achieve what l would like with the talent l had. If it hadn't been for the phlebotomy l would have probably succeeded.

I don't know if l knew what period l lived in. No, not really, I don't think l did. But l had only the faintest idea of the human tragedy that was unfolding before me. Domestic scenes from a Pinter play. Simple and epic. Mother had long been literally annihilated. When l was six she was dragged off to the 'care' of the mental 'health' services where l was consequently to see her only very rarely. My father's ingenious violence led her to a spectacular form of emotional distress and suffering that marked my young mind and shaped me for the future. My own deep emotional distress was so easy for my father to provoke. This is with what l grew up. Absence and violence. These where my only references. My father's complacent bonhomie with other coppers allowed a comprehensive neglect of his youngest from a very early age without ever being investigated by the social services. He had only the faintest conscience of his thorough negligence and as far as providing an education was completely devoid of means or capacity. My father's language was as brutal as any of his blows. Although l have suffered with my children, l have tried to communicate with them.

After this failure of any effective familial education l was left to fend for myself from a very early age. I knew what the violence of being abandoned meant at the age of six. I tried to form extra household relationships with friends with which l had only limited empathy. I used narcotics at the age of fifteen mostly to bond with a supposed tribe, which simply didn't exist. I wonder when things got out of hand? At the age of seventeen. I had used LSD or rather was coerced into using it and poisoned by it. My handle on reality dwindled and then was mostly a vague memory.

My distress was immediately treated with what are dangerous chemicals, without once asking me what happened to me. They said l had a biological disease of the brain. Not once has someone suggested to me that l should withdraw. I became a living taboo. A sacrificial totem for unsaid abuse with no way out, as l was seen as mentally ill. I believe there is a great amount of money to be made by forcing these drugs on those of us who are most vulnerable. It's an ascendancy that the white clothed 'carers' enjoy because it enables them to torment their victims with a good conscience. Torture.

My imposed position has adversely affected everyone around me. I never knew that it could be possible to be so alone. That one could be so isolated, lonely. As if everyone had disappeared. Lost to familiar surroundings, to no longer belong. I never knew it was possible to feel such a feeling of loss, fear and abandonment. Suddenly there I was in the middle of this. I was not bleeding, but I was trapped … to resignation and a morose resolve. I sometimes think of acting out, as a kind of revenge for the smug and delusional arrogance of the shrinks, or for the hypocrisy of the nurses. I sometimes imagined taking revenge. But I wouldn't do it. I feel calmed by these thoughts at times, as if they were natural, though I know there is nothing natural about this situation.

It is a soluble dissolution of a life. Irredeemably and irrevocably that which l am not; neither chosen or desired, but imposed. This was the worst of it. Looking back, the incomprehension. I would have gladly paid for any error l made, and leave it at that, but this was to go so much further. Perhaps l committed an error, something stupid or dumb of which l was unaware. But this could never be paid for entirely. Soljenitsyne describes the use of neuroleptics as torture. My experience of them is the meaning of the word.

My so called family, which consisted uniquely of my father at that time, did not take the least interest in who l was or what l was doing. Not once did my father have any curiosity in the work l was supposed to be doing at school. My brothers had left the house years ago, and they were too occupied trying to earn a living than to worry what their much younger brother was doing. l didn't see it coming.

I had an English teacher, Miss B, who warned me about the dangers of cannabis when l was fifteen. There was the religious education teacher, Mr P, who gave a very brief description of the dangers of certain drugs, and that was it.

Naïveté: my youthful years and tremendous isolation meant that l wished badly to be one of the crowd. I took different narcotics in order to blend in and to bond with the other pupils who were experimenting with dangerous substances. Then one day, imbibed onto a square of blotting paper, was some Lysergic Acid Diethylamide offered to me as a kind of initiation. It was this poison that led to my first bout of extreme emotional distress.

With the weight of my past, with its pitiless abuse of many kinds, things got out of hand and l couldn't function in the sparse social context l found myself in. There were behavioural difficulties and incoherence that made it clear l wasn't able to cope alone, a situation l had been in since the internment, and subsequent absence of my mother many years beforehand.

I was locked away from public scrutiny. Forcibly sedated as l have been to this day.

I was lucky not to have ECT administered like my mother whose death from a massive brain haemorrhage was a direct result of the torture. She received fourteen series of ECT which fragilised her cerebral blood vessels that led to her death after this barbaric chemical and electric torture. l could never have known the extent of her torture or what she had to go through cut off, as she was, from her three children. Towards the end she had manifest brain damage, her memory was as frail as her physical condition, her speech was slurred and her eyesight bad. She had seen so much abuse, from the entry into Berlin of the Russians in 1945, four soldiers raping her at the age of fifteen, to her imprisonment in Broadmoor for years with the entailing torture that is practiced there. I loved her every bit as she loved me. She was an authentic combatant in a war of high intensity. I seek her revenge. l remember our visits to Broadmoor. It is a barbaric place with no dignity. I remember the noise of the keys of the locks that were everywhere. I had a glimpse of what awaited me in France years later. That these places still exist is a damning indictment to obligatory medical 'protocols' and the lack of any effective alternatives. They just satisfy themselves with masturbatory discourses and biased science that schizophrenia is a brain disease which is characterized by too much dopamine in the post synapses. As if they knew when they first developed neuroleptics: they knew nothing then, they know nothing now.

- when l think of it now, I tell myself that people are very fragile. An identity. This fragility is striking. This sureness that can break so quickly and fall. You're there, living and becoming. You're there with your promise contained within, your dreams, your desires. Then, for you, it's finished. All the promise you contained vanishes. You contain no longer anything, not one promise. One day you've achieved nothing. This is what happens to you. This is what you become. Someone who has achieved nothing, done nothing.

- And the passage is very rapid. Just before it happens you're still in the realm of possibilities, what could become. Then afterwards, just after, it's finished. After there is no longer anything left that's possible. And that's the only thing that is left, an absence of possibilities.

- (The doubtful man).

Edward Walter is the pen name of John Herbert.
I have grappled with emotional distress since 1979 when l was 17 years old. This distress has had serious consequences. Am a lover of nature and reading, two interests which provide me with a semblance of freedom.

Of All Things
A Collection of Poems
Bridget Conway

November 8, 2012

The gassy smelling air on the cool wind in late spring
I don't know why the few people who do love me, love me
So I wither in dust and guilt and messy hair piled up on brick shaped
skies

June 3, 2015

Today is as gloomy as the next
The light shines on my afternoon cheeks as a reminder that I've done
nothing yet
With a heavy head I lean towards the window and whisper breaths
untwined
When will you stop and leave me alone?
I unhinge my door with sore bones
And push open the world in front of me
Too much
Too soon

June 16, 2015

I had the thought
Of passing on
Into a realm of nothing

A land oblivious of time
But then I woke to the sun pouring into my cave
I wondered then
Where there and here begins

August 23, 2015

I claw at the open wounds of the world
The clouds pulse with the scraping sounds of the inside of my skull
And I echoed on a Sunday
The same old song
The same old me
Learning to be free
And living in between

November 5, 2015

On those days when everything feels heavy
There is nothing that can be done
To lighten a load that shutters itself inside your mind
Except to escape your mind completely
Go out of it
Leave it on the desk
Cut it up on the chopping board
Let it spill over
Onto the dirty floor

November 10, 2015

Just let me keep track
Of my own bruises on my own time
I will count them on the precipice of the highest
And coldest place
Way up in the crying clouds
They are sad
Because we make them different than what they want to be
And they weep until
My wounds become ghosts

February 2, 2016

I've lived for months
Amidst the bustling crowd
Of sky-high towers and shining lights
Yet a calm centre
Breeding happiness within
I've learned to deal
With all the storms that try to break in

March 9, 2016

When you count days
Like each one will hang you
Out on a limb in the void of memory
Then it's been 365 days of forgetting
One year ago I arrived
Inside my mind and sat down

With every fibre of my mouth, I spoke
Words of sadness and destruction
It was time to begin the journey
Which would lead me to today

December 6, 2018

These hands
Open to the sky
Rain pours and floods inside my mind
This experience
Of all things
Is the strength beneath my heart
It's purpose standing tall
A breath goes inwards
And out to the unforgiving
Limitless night
The moon carries my weight
And she spins

Bridget is a social worker, nerd, and cat lady. She experienced a lot of trauma while growing up in America. In 2015, she tried to end her life, only to end up in the 'system'. Poetry allows her to express herself; she wouldn't be where she is today without it.

Screening for psychosis and finding a person
James Rylan

Psychosis has a particular purpose for me and it's not the same meaning that clinicians refer to. Clinicians talk about bizarre behaviour, for me I'm focussing on something that has my attention. The way I see the experience of psychosis is that it helped me survive some painful events in my life. As a child, I didn't know what good coping was. I come from a culture that respects elders, childhood sexual, verbal or emotional abuse wasn't talked about. But this is what I experienced. The racing thoughts and dissociation that I experienced as an adolescent took some of the pain away. Having the same symptoms unravel as an adult helped me survive thoughts and feelings that were attached to the past, a time that is too difficult to accept. As an adult, I was too unwell to think clearly which disrupted my day to day activities.

Psychosis at its peak stops you from getting into clean clothes, having a shower, eating and making contact with friends or acquaintances. It takes you away from work. Memory loss, disorganised thinking and delusions impact your relationships and the physical environment you live in. Attempts at tidying up results in me walking around my house and being heavily distracted. Psychosis in moderation is purposeful, full blown and you need external help. The help I have had for psychosis has been tremendous, slow but really helpful. Ironically the psychiatrists don't ask whether it's ok to take away my symptoms. Through involuntary restraint they decide that they will take away my symptoms, symptoms that probably kept me alive during the vulnerable periods of my life.

Some days and some of the time, in my day to day life, I have to challenge thoughts that lead me to feel like 'I'm doing the wrong thing'. These thoughts creep up when I'm eating, about to purchase groceries. When the thought is strong, I will put back the item and leave the shop without buying what I needed, I will stop eating. I'll be ready to leave my house, then the thoughts get in my way. Sometimes I drink to get rid of the them. Luckily, I'm a lot more competent in leaving the house now than I was a few months ago. These thoughts fluctuate in their intensity. When I'm really excited the thoughts go away and I'm free to wonder the world.

Things that I have found helpful in my journey:

Supported Employment

One of the first helpful supports I had was supported employment. I was initially rejected for this as I didn't have a Centrelink payment. I didn't even know about Centrelink payments. The disability support pension (DSP) opened up the opportunity for a job and to get references, which I didn't have. I was hired on a cleaning crew. We had early 8am starts. I was a good worker, but one morning I called in sick, I didn't have a medical certificate and thought I would get fired. I was too anxious to answer any of their phone calls and so that was the end of supported employment for me. What I hadn't grasped was that I wouldn't have been fired, I would have been supported and progressed in my employment. The impacts of my anxiety and how I understand got in the way. I later heard that I was one of the all-time best workers. Had I known this while I was working, I wouldn't have taken a day off. I can work through this next time by approaching, rather than avoiding, anxious situations.

Working in Partners in Recovery (PIR)

I interviewed successfully to get a job in the PIR program. This was my first successful job interview. PIR focusses on the individual and system levels of consumer service journey making sure people are connected to suitable services and services are focussed on the individual's needs. This was a program close to my heart given the negative experiences that I had had with services and being able to provide opportunities to people I worked with.

Independence, Connection, Purpose and Meaning

The best I have ever been was after a trip overseas. I stopped taking the medications that had been prescribed for me as I didn't want to explain these to border security nor my family that I was travelling with. When I came back, I was soo relaxed that I didn't resume the meds. I had a full-time job and played soccer, I was living in a shared house which started off with four flatmates and when I moved out 10 people were living there. The supports of work, accommodation, making friends and activity in playing soccer really helped to keep symptoms from returning.

Hospital

My best friend is from hospital. When all I can succeed in is walking around inside my house, hospital seems like an okay place to be. My admissions have been involuntary – for behaviour, hypomanic episode, malnutrition and psychosis. I've had some awesome doctors, and some that forget patients are people.

Public Mental Health Service and Community Treatment Order (CTO)

For a short period of time I secretly liked being on a CTO. Given my history with services, where I either couldn't get help or my thoughts were too disorganised to stay in touch, the CTO enabled consistent access to a caring mental health service.

The CTO wasn't able to help me stay well in the community. The service prioritised symptom control over my own goals and some of my needs. I was too anxious to go into the centre in order to meet the requirements of the CTO. I am anxious to visit mental health sites due to an experience I had where I was strip searched with multiple nurses and security guards watching. None of them were on my side. I was shaking and felt like I was watching myself. Back to the CTO – not having made a psychiatrist appointment nor attending the centre for medication administration meant I had breached the CTO which led to another two-month hospitalisation. Once again, I missed three months of full-time work and income.

In addition to refusing medication, I believe I ended up on a CTO as I was not forthcoming of how aware I was with my symptoms. This led me to fall into the lack of insight category. From my experience crisis teams and hospital deciding that I need help means I get the help that I need, compared to the closed door that I could get if I self-presented or specified that I needed support.

When the CTO ended the service would follow up with me unlike voluntary services where, if the consumer didn't make contact, the service would assume that support was no longer wanted or needed, although the real reason for lack of contact could be paranoia, trouble organising a contact time, fear, disordered thinking or past experiences with services. The service has now started home visits. A year ago, I wouldn't have consented to home visits to avoid a negative experience in my house. For now, home visits are working well.

A service following up makes it real – is nice and humane.

Peer Transitional Service

Through the hospital I was connected to a short-term peer support service. I was also referred to a couple of NGOs (non-government organisations) with whom I lost contact easily. Peer Support has been one of the best services that I have engaged with. I can laugh with the peer worker and he meets me in places where I am comfortable. He has been a bridge in filling in gaps between me and the mental health service. He's really helpful.

Getting the diagnosis of Bipolar Disorder and Treatment Resistant Schizophrenia

I was initially given the diagnosis of Borderline Personality Disorder (BPD) and with it came multiple closed doors to my attempts at figuring out what was going on for me. I was self-harming, a female who wanted to die without having a reason for that. This combination would be seen as typical of BPD. I applied for a case manager to help me with concentration and getting my Uni work done. (This was something I was really struggling to get ahead on, and really what could I have expected when my headspace was filled with anxiety?) I was declined for case management and advised that my concerns (i.e. BPD) could be better helped by a private psychologist. So, I had asked for help years before my experiences escalated to psychosis, and I was declined help. And here I am years later forced to have case management which comes with a CTO.

Oh man!

It brings a smile to my face.

I'm a student. I'm very interested in getting involved in having my say in shaping mental health services. I would really like services to respond faster, be consistent, follow up and use technology to help with social interaction and communication difficulties that may impact on engagement with a service. I am proud of achieving a degree in neuroscience.

Embracing My Authentic Self
Vicki Katsifis

Emotional distress and extreme states have produced a powerful personal transformation of my sense of self – from a shattered, fragile shell to a strong authentic self.

I believe that emotional distress is an attempt by the mind and body to heal something that has happened to us rather than simply a biochemical condition that has no root or cause. Without these experiences I wouldn't have explored my self-concept and transformed it.

I have been able to integrate my childhood with the assistance of an extreme state, and heal from grief and loss.

My workplace and participation in the mental health advocacy movement helped me rebuild my confidence. Love and connection to central people in my life gave me a space to grow my authenticity and true essence, which provided a firm foundation of self.

Growing up Greek was particularly difficult for me as I didn't have a strong bond with my mother. My mother had some health concerns and was a very quiet person. She faded into the background in my childhood whilst my brother, father and I had a tight bond. My father was larger-than-life and I was extremely close to him. This lack of attachment to my mother affected me quite deeply. It was very hard to live up to the Greek cultural norms of having all the necessary skills to be a good Greek housewife, pivotal to a woman's role in my culture. I longed to learn those skills but with the lack of a maternal bond, this proved very difficult. I also felt I needed guidance in how to be feminine and to fit into the Greek culture.

This led to a fragile sense of self where my only sense of competency was in the world of academia and studying. Whenever I visited relatives, I felt very insecure and different to my female cousins who were very adept at being good Greek girls. This significantly impacted my self-concept, and view of myself as a worthwhile person.

Being labelled with a diagnosis affected me deeply and contributed to my lack of selfhood. I became a shell of my former self and felt isolated and separate from the rest of society. I remember walking the streets of my neighbourhood and feeling different from the members of my community. I sensed a degree of separation with everybody else as though a mark on my forehead had labelled me deficient and not worthy of love and connection.

When I was nineteen years of age, my father died of a heart attack in his sleep. This was sudden and very shocking to me. We were so close: I felt utterly bereft, isolated and alone.

In my interaction with public mental health services I truly believed that my grief and loss issues concerning my father, and my lack of a secure sense of self would be addressed. I felt that somebody would ask me what had happened to me. I was quickly labelled and diagnosed with a mental health condition and fed a vast variety of drugs. There was no counselling over my significant loss, and nobody I could talk to.

I have always felt that my extreme states have been very symbolic, and a powerful part of my healing journey.

During these states I have been able to develop deep insights into my family situation and have had moments when previously repressed emotions were unleashed. The content of these experiences was often metaphorical and symbolic to my history. Once I reached a level of wellness and distance from these states, I was able to acknowledge the healing messages they provided and integrate them.

One extreme state gifted me with a strong feeling of love and peace in myself, that I am still able to access to this day.

During this state, I felt a spiritual presence that offered me warmth, love, acceptance and wisdom. This presence felt very maternal and I was able to construct a dialogue where I could ask questions about my life situation and intuit a response that was wise, warm and healing. Whilst this dialogue was engendered during an extreme state, in my current state of wellness through prayer and reflection, I am still able to facilitate this loving healing energy. It provides me with answers to issues I'm grappling with. This spiritual connection can be labelled and diagnosed, but I feel it lovingly gives me something that I felt was lacking in my childhood – and a connection I truly yearned for. It gifts me with a strong, loving maternal presence. It helps me feel connected to something larger than myself, to heal my feelings of abandonment and grief and loss. It is an anchor that assists me to feel strong and secure.

I have had some wonderful opportunities in my workplaces to rebuild my identity. In one job my manager entrusted me with a project to deliver on Work, Health and Safety which would provide accreditation for our service. I had no knowledge of this area but she fully believed that I could do it. This unwavering belief in my ability to manage the project and bring it to fruition, gave me the positive reinforcement that I lacked in childhood. Being put into challenging situations by people who believed in me, and having the resolve to move through them, has been life changing.

In my current role I was given the chance to be acting manager of the organisation. This was very daunting as I felt I was not decisive enough for the position. I was able to develop strategies to move through my anxieties and performed decisively and effectively. Having my manager strongly believe that I had the skills, attributes and capabilities to do the role, gave me a platform to develop my burgeoning sense of self and transform it into a strong one.

People and connections facilitated my transformation. After a few extreme states, many people in my life had abandoned me, and were not interested in resuming connections. My best friend since primary school reconnected with me after my diagnosis and offered her friendship and support at a time when I was isolated and alone. She has diligently stood beside me through all my ups and downs, and offered me a consistent long-term friendship. Through my extreme states she would patiently wait for the state to dissipate and then resume the friendship. She would declare to others that I was her best friend. This declaration was powerful as it gave me personal value and contributed to a stronger foundation.

My brother was also able to see that I was a worthwhile person – who would one day heal – and he accepted me completely. He would affirm to me that my extreme states were an expression of something deeper and not the totality of who I was as a person. He included me in his circle of friends and felt proud of me at a time when not many people were around.

Falling in love is a wonderful healer. Losing my father and receiving a diagnosis impacted my health significantly. Meeting my partner and having someone walk beside me in my journey, has accelerated my healing. He acts as a daily sounding board, and by articulating my deep-seated issues to him, there is an impetus to make the commitment to resolving them. He motivates me to develop my own strategies to cope and helps me explore the significance and meaning of my experiences. He offers me a safe place to land, and an abiding love.

Embracing my authentic self has been transformative for me. Throughout my life, I have often felt overwhelmed by other people's needs and wants, and had weak boundaries. I practice authenticity with my partner daily, and with his support, love and encouragement, my true self filters through all my other relationships. To be proud and speak my truth is extremely powerful and healing.

I find solidarity and passion in the mental health advocacy movement. Being a part of something larger than myself: striving for people who experience emotional distress to be viewed as equal, contributing members of society, who are simply responding to something significant that has happened to them, rather than a pathology, is what gives my life drive, meaning, and purpose.

Forming a strong bond with my mother has been part of my healing journey. I deepened our relationship by listening to her life story and sharing mine with her during weekly outings. We slowly got closer and have a unique understanding of each other's life. This has been a true gift for me.

Emotional distress is a signal, warning us of something deeper at play. My emotional distress was crying out to me that I needed to urgently work on my sense of self. My extreme states led me to a sense of spirituality and powerful healing, and the support emanating from love, friendship, family, my workplace, and the mental health advocacy movement, allowed me to embrace my authentic self.

Vicki has worked in the mental health sector for over twenty years in roles including peer work, consumer advocacy, multicultural mental health, the non-government field and in peer education. Vicki is passionate about people healing from their mental health issue by discovering what has happened to them rather than looking at what is wrong with them. She believes people need to make meaning out of what has happened and discover their authenticity and true voice.

A Stranger I Remain
John

My story begins when I was fourteen years old, when I had my first psychotic break. Quite frankly I didn't know what was happening to me, it was as if my mind and my body were disagreeing as to what was happening to me.

My body was telling me that everything was fine and nothing was going on but my mind was telling me that it was all going to hell in a handbasket and I needed to escape and run from everyone and everything. I ended up having to go to hospital with my mother and my sister, who were an absolute rock during this ordeal. This ordeal lasted over twelve hours and I was sent home after I had been given some medication to calm me down.

Fast forward to when I was eighteen, I had another psychotic break, this one being so severe that I needed to be put in the mental health unit at the local hospital. I was terrified throughout the whole time I was there as being admitted to hospital was one of my greatest fears. I was hospitalised for a total of four days and that is when I was put on medication on a regular basis.

After this I was linked to the local mental health service. I will be the first to admit that I had feelings of trepidation, cynicism and worry. What I worried about most was "Will they judge me for how I look, act or speak". My mother and my sister both assured me that no matter what happened I would not be judged in any way shape or form. I usually hate to admit when I am wrong but in this case I am happy to say that I was dead wrong.

I was pleasantly surprised with how accepting they were of me and my issues.

It was at a psychiatrist's appointment that I was told about a few of my issues. At first, I was scared that those issues would define me but it was my mother who said, "the names of those issues are nothing but words and they do not define who you are or what you can do". She jumped on to the internet and pulled up list after list of people who had the same issues I have.

Almost one year to the day later was my second hospitalisation; again I had the feelings of fear, being terrified, but most of all I felt an overwhelming feeling of disassociation. It was as if I could see, feel and hear what was going on but it felt like I was just going through the motions, almost as if nothing felt real. I was in hospital for a grand total of seven days. My meds were adjusted.

It was after the second hospitalisation that I really started to find my footing and accepted the fact that I was not what society deemed "normal". My mother and my sister said it best and often, that "normal is nothing more than a setting on a washing machine but even then washing machines are losing that setting."

An unexpected consequence of all this was that no matter hard I tried, no matter how much I wanted to, I could never see myself the same way I used to. I guess the reason why is because I knew I was different but I never wanted to admit to myself or others through fear of rejection or alienation.

With hindsight I can see that the reason I was feeling this way is because

I didn't understand how many people were going through something similar. I didn't want to be the only one going through this, but through my own research I quickly discovered that I was not alone and that many people have gone through or were going through their own journey that was similar yet completely different to mine.

Soon after this I was introduced to my case manager who in turn put me in contact with my psychologist and other services. By talking with my psychologist, we came up with strategies to help combat the negative sides of potential relapses. My case manager organised for me to see a psychiatrist. The psychiatrist spoke to me with regards to my diagnosis and asked how I felt about it all. At first, I didn't want to believe it was true, I didn't want to tell anyone or let anyone close enough know because of the stigma attached to mental health.

Over time my psychologist and I worked out a plethora of strategies that when used correctly, helped me to truly understand that my diagnosis was nothing more than words on a piece of paper and that is was up to me if I let it define me and let it hang over me like a rock hanging precariously off a cliff. I made the choice to not let that rock fall and follow the path of my journey.

At first, I thought that my journey would be as smooth as skating on an ice skating rink. There is only one problem with that analogy: I don't know how to ice skate so my journey has been full of dizzying highs and troublesome lows but the only way to keep going with my journey was to keep getting up, working my way through barriers in my way.

I would like to give special thanks to my mother and sister, who have been there for me since this all started. I would also like to thank my psychologist for being the utmost professional, and my case manager who knew when to keep it serious but also when to lighten the mood.

In summary, I still have my defence mechanisms up, and yes I have trouble breaking them down. Slowly but surely, I will get to where I want to be and continue on with my plans to have a healthy, happy and fulfilling life because let's face it, what is considered normal?

My name is John and I am in the midst of my mental health journey. While writing this piece I am trying to help bring more awareness and understanding of mental health also I am trying to break the stigma attached to mental health.

Scars Are Maps Of Who You Are
Melissa Asta

I didn't know where the urge came from. I'd never felt it before, but it was too big to ignore. To not follow through was not an option. So, I picked up a piece of the glass I'd just thrown across the room and buried it into my skin.

I was 19 the first time I cut myself. The idea of doing something like this to myself had never occurred to me before. I had never known anyone who had done it and I'd never really heard of the concept.

I had been medicated for depression since I was 12 years old. The depression had been attributed to the Chronic Fatigue Syndrome I'd been diagnosed with at the same age. However, it wasn't until I had a hormone implant inserted to treat endometriosis that I really felt I'd lost control.

My mood was lower than it had ever been but it manifested itself as anger. I began to verbally lash out at my family and my boyfriend. This was extremely unlike me. At the time I was very reserved, shy and had difficulty asserting myself in any way. I had never even 'talked back' to my parents in my life so this was incredibly out of character.

I felt this massive surge of emotion growing inside me. Anger, sadness, fear, frustration, confusion all melded together to create this overwhelming pressure that I could feel somatically. It became more than just the emotion, it felt like a physical growth, a tumour, the cells of which multiplied by the second and my body could no longer contain it. I had to get 'it' out and yelling and screaming just were not providing the kind of relief I needed. I needed release and my instinct was to create it an exit.

The release, relief, was instantaneous. Like I'd found a pressure valve. I sank onto the kitchen floor and felt all of the intensity melt away. My mind calmed and my muscles relaxed. I felt almost 'normal' again.

I thought then that what had happened was a freak incident, a one-off, something that transpired in that moment of overwhelm, but the hormone implant couldn't be removed and I had to wait for it to dissolve. As such, all those feelings would inevitably make themselves too big for my body to confine and now I had discovered the most effective remedy.

Along with the release, cutting myself brought on feelings of elation. It boosted my mood. I felt a buzz, like I was high and I would talk a million miles a minute. It felt like I could have fun again, I could be happy, I could feel free.

With time, the side effects of the implant wore off and life went back to, well, a new kind of normal. Yes, I was back at work. No, I wasn't becoming blindingly angry at a moment's notice and taking it out on the people who meant the most to me. Yet, I was somehow more fragile. I was aware that people regarded me differently, almost fearfully. Back then, self-harm was rarely heard of. The visible scarring did not help.

Eventually, the anti-depressant medication I had continued to take wasn't keeping me well any more. The old pressure built up on its own without requiring the fuel of the hormones and I began applying my most effective feel-good measure on a daily basis, several times a day.

I did seek help. I knew how these measures made me feel, but during the come down from my high, I was also acutely aware of the effect of these

measures on those closest to me. I saw their tears while they patched me up, felt their fear that this was the pre-cursor to suicide. I was never left alone. The kitchen knives were suddenly nowhere to be found.
So, I looked for help.

I called helplines, triage services, had visits from the crisis assessment team. I kept up with my meds and my doctor's appointments. I had numerous hospital admissions, endured many courses of Electro-Convulsive Therapy (ECT), and visits to emergency to have myself stitched up. Even with all of this (and more that I haven't mentioned) no one could suggest anything that would help me feel better faster than cutting myself. Things like flicking a rubber band against my wrist or dripping red food dye on my arm were never going to cut it. So to speak.

No one could help me because no one could understand why I was doing it or how I could find something so destructive, so beneficial.

I began to lose friends because they couldn't fathom why I was engaging in this behaviour and why I wouldn't just stop. It wasn't only those close to me who were not equipped to handle this. Even some medical professionals from whom I sought assistance were not kind. One emergency department (ED) nurse said I shouldn't need a local anaesthetic when she stitched my wound. On another occasion in ED, a doctor with psychiatric experience said to me, "Why should I help you? You did this to yourself."

The strange thing is, the cutting itself was never really painful. For me, it wasn't primarily about converting emotional pain into physical pain in an effort to control it. It was all about that release. Eventually, the blood I lost became a physical representation of that release – the more I bled, the more relief I felt. The scratches I started with were no longer sufficient and I regularly needed stitches.

Something else that added to my cravings for self-harm was the, admittedly, sad sense of pride I gleaned from the act. No one else I knew did this, *could* do this. I convinced myself that being able to do it meant I was strong. It gave me a sense of achievement. I'd had to leave my job in Melbourne and move back to Central Victoria so I was closer to the support of family. To me, this meant I had failed at life. Cutting was something I could do and I was good at it.

It is important to acknowledge two things: first, that self-harm is rarely a suicide attempt; second, that the majority of those who self-harm have experienced trauma of some description in their lifetime. For people who have been diagnosed with Borderline Personality Disorder (or preferably Complex Trauma Disorder as some wonderfully empathetic professionals are attempting to have it re-classified) and for which self-harm is a dominant symptom, 75 per cent (and some have said even up to 80-90 per cent) are survivors of childhood trauma. And yet self-harm is often attributed to 'attention-seeking'. If so many of us have survived such extremes, what if this is a factor that contributes to keeping us alive?

I am now employed as a Peer Support Worker in a short term residential mental health facility. In my two and a half years working there, probably the most difficult question I've been asked is "How can I stop self-harming?" When someone asks me this question it feels physically painful because I know exactly how it feels to ask that question, the pain and desperation it requires, but predominantly because I know I don't have a definitive answer.

I can end this piece by saying that I do not cut myself any more. As of the time of writing, it has been 524 days since I last intentionally drew my own blood. That is, by far, the longest period I have gone without cutting since that very first time. The only other time that has come close is when I vowed to myself that I wouldn't self-harm while I was pregnant with my son. I will not say that the urge is gone because I would be lying if I did, but now I know, in no uncertain terms, that I will not follow through.

The reason is this: For the 30 years that I was contending with my mental illness, my biggest question was, "Why?" "Why was I so unwell?" "Why was my potential being squandered?" "Why was my life such a waste?" I tried to be content with the 'chemical imbalance' theory, that this was 'just how I was'. It wasn't until I felt safe enough to allow myself to acknowledge my trauma, and to face it head on, that my healing began. I will not lie and say it has been easy, or quick. I know this will be something I will have to work at for many years. However, it will be, and is, worth it.

And I will never ever let the perpetrators of that trauma leave another scar on my body.

I am Melissa. I am mother to a wonderfully weird 10-year-old boy, Eli, and partner to the most patient man on earth, Joel. I am lucky enough to be a Peer Worker which I absolutely love, attempting to make something good out of my bad.

For Violet
Ella

The information came as a wonderful and timely revelation and I could breathe again! I was excited and relieved to have found an explanation for madness that actually matched my experience. It ended months of misery and swept away my suicide plan.

It was 1994 and I had been experiencing tough circumstances and irreconcilable conflicts, which led to my third, week-long episode of psychosis. My threshold to psychosis had probably been lowered by childhood experiences and some unusual intergenerational trauma and injustice on all sides of the family. I was brought up in a family who, in those days, readily took on the interchangeable roles of victim, rescuer and persecutor. This became my way of being in the world.

During the episode I behaved extremely badly... believing that I was helping or rescuing people. If I hadn't been mad/psychotic, I would have ended up in the criminal justice system. (Fortunately, my behaviour in this antidepressant-induced episode was never repeated).

I was hospitalised for the first time. The father of my eighteen month daughter required me to sign custody consent papers before I could see my daughter. Close friends were wonderful, but my appalling behaviour, custody loss, 'treatment' and negative social status, led to a sense of shame, defectiveness and despair.

Several dismal months down the post-diagnosis road, my body bloated by lithium, a friend handed me a book by Arnold Mindell. The book contained case studies of a Process Work approach to extreme states... and led to the epiphany I mentioned in the beginning.

After finishing the book, I awoke next morning with the sensations of vibration, lightness, space between my cells and a feeling of peace and aliveness. This three day experience helped to re-establish my bearings in life.

It made sense that I had been overwhelmed by circumstances and needed to change certain beliefs and life situations in order to cope. My usual personality disintegrated in order to reintegrate differently. Some 'not-me', aspects of myself and others around me were needed. These lesser known aspects were given a chance to drive the collective bus of my psyche... something for which they had little training, experience or support to do. My socially-adapted aspects were asleep down the back of the bus. Neither group was talking with the other.

From Mindell's book I recognised that I had been acting in the world while my mind had been Dreaming. I learnt that such an awareness/ growth process can be supported and fulfilled... or interrupted, thwarted, or frozen and perhaps recycled in a more difficult way. Also, that madness/'the problem' does not reside solely within an individual but exists beyond and between people, and is cultural.

I was primed to embrace these positive ideas due to my two previous episodes. My first episode occurred in 1987 at the age of 32. Accurate telepathy suddenly opened up – which was quite astonishing and led to a blissful form of 'Unitive Consciousness'. Outcomes included embracing my female identity – no longer believing that females were inferior and less wanted than males. I also began a reconciliation with my mother from whom I had become estranged in early childhood.

During a second episode in 1989, I stopped speaking and discovered among other interesting things that I could play the piano with my own music and pick up the guitar and make up songs.

The biological, biochemical explanation cannot account for these things. A process approach does – while still being compatible with medication that is helpful for so many of us.

Process (rather than state-based) responses were not available for me, and nor were they for Violet.

In 1930's New Zealand at the age of 42, Violet Annette Webb had a gynaecological operation with a chloroform anaesthetic. She awoke in an altered reality and saw snakes climbing up the walls and spiders crawling over her bed. Three days later she was put in a locked room in a psychiatric hospital, given painful, repetitive shock treatment, and remained there until her death 35 years later.

Such fearful haste to bring my grandmother back to consensus reality by force had devastating consequences over time. It seemed that someone in our family needed to sift through the ashes of her experience in order to find any jewel of value for us today.

At thirteen, when I learnt that my grandmother had lived in a psychiatric hospital, I immediately decided that I must hide my 'sensitive strangeness' and avoid bringing attention to myself – or I would be put away for the rest of my life too. Thanks to that unworkable decision, I unwittingly volunteered to sift through the ashes.

Whenever I share Violet's story with others, people usually respond with, "Oh, but it's so much better these days". I reply, "Yes and NO!" The dominant viewpoint (from which the treatments of the day arise) is identical. Rather than an appreciation of something challenging but valuable trying to happen, there is the same limited interpretation – of a wrongness/illness, to be crushed.

It really concerns me that there is a teaching within psychiatry that any time spent in psychosis causes brain damage and a kindling of further episodes. Except possibly for a psychosis of longer than ninety days, this myth derives from a single, flawed research paper – and is used to legitimise immediate drug suppression. Ample research exists including controlled trials (sidelined by the psychiatric industry) showing that people who don't receive anti-psychotic drugs during an episode usually do significantly better in the longer term. *(References to this can be found in a book by Professor of Psychiatry, George McCouch[1].)*

Even before discovering this information, I was compelled to achieve what Violet was denied. I looked for supportive supervision during an episode, and so I became a kind of (socially alarming) guinea pig in my own experiment.

Further profound altered states occurred over the following years. I typically walked around naked in public and in many of the episodes believed I was dead. I was hospitalised many times. People with far heavier trauma than myself can experience psychosis as a nightmare of extreme fear and suffering but my distress happened before and afterwards.

---

1 *George McCouch, (2018), "While Psychiatry Slept – Reawakening the Imagination in the Therapeutic Process", Santa Fe, Belly Song Press, pp. 81-82.*

Many years, adventures and disasters later, at long last I was fully supervised by friends over the week of an episode. Naked, I sang with a new voice, laughed, played and clowned around. Eleven friends supported at different times, and I found it especially wonderful to be joined by some of them in what I was doing. The episode ended well, without hospitalisation.

Something important released in me thanks to being 'met' in all my madness. The angry emotionality of the mission I had been undertaking transformed into a more gentle purpose.

After that, in a way that surprised people, I became willing to take medication whenever necessary so as not to take risks anymore – I need to take it rarely and briefly. I don't want to worry the people around me or ask for time and attention from friends in that way again, and alternative sanctuary care (eg Diabasis, i Ward, Soteria) is unavailable in Australia.

I became involved in the Australian Spiritual Emergence Network (SEN). This organisation provides support resources for people who experience Extreme States. I was particularly drawn to SEN because Spiritual, Transpersonal, Existential and Paranormal experiences are usually missing from other approaches.

Despite misrepresentations Spiritual Emergency is not a stand-alone concept, rather it is holistic and exists alongside physical, psychological and social dimensions. (Causation can be due to poisoning, brain tumours, drugs etc. Resolution may involve dealing with trauma, relationship and social issues.)

I studied Process Oriented Psychology (Process Work) over seven years and do my best to practise this in my life. Arnold Mindell and colleagues developed this as a progression of Jung's work. Attention is given to incorporating the Dreaming dimension, and it makes my heart sing. 'The Dreaming', as I use the term, refers to that which is trying to emerge into our awareness that is unknown, denied or rejected. The Dreaming reveals itself in disturbances, our bodies, emotions, social interactions, the physical world, the numinous, and the dreams of sleep.

Despite these influences, for many years I worried about the perspective that western society insisted I adopt. Did I really have a defective brain and a bi-polar 'mental illness'? I began listening to the archive list of speakers on www.madnessradio.net and was inspired by the wide range of professionals who work beyond the medical model. Months later I realised that the subtle, illness-identity depression that I had worn around myself like a cloak, had vanished.

Although I have been stable for many years, I am cautious of my vulnerability, and still have a long way to go with confidence, work and being fully present. More lightly now, I remain dedicated to achieving respectful responses to people in profound altered states – responses which involve, amongst other things, following and supporting the Dreaming process as a guide through crisis.

Ella Linwood (born 1955) is from Aotearoa-New Zealand, and lives in Maleny, Queensland. She especially enjoys life with her husband, daughter, wider family, friends and cat. She also enjoys gardening, nature, music, languages, comedy and a whole lot of other things. Information about Ella's work can be found on her website: www.grounding-dreaming.net

Black Birds
Kylie Gyaneshwar

With the clarity of hindsight, I believe I've lived with mental illness for most of my life. I had panic attacks as a child, nightmares, and many fears. Through adolescence there were, of course, events in varying shades of the traumatic that would send my mental health spiraling, such as my parents' divorce, and the culture shock of moving to a new country where I felt foreign and culturally illiterate. I went through puberty, racism, a painful relationship with my father, a struggle with my cultural identity, and feelings of displacement. But all of these things seemed somehow normal parts of life. Things many teenagers were living with. My extreme level of distress at times didn't feel warranted or justified. I now know that back then I was, at times, deeply depressed and emotionally distressed. I thought often of suicide.

Only recently a psychiatrist told me my symptoms were consistent with Dysthymic Disorder, a chronic low-level form of depression, with episodes of major depression. This is how my life has felt. Mostly struggling through the days feeling low with rare moments when I could say I truly felt good. Enduring life rather than living it.

Feeling invisible, unable to make meaningful friendships amongst the social whirl of university, I had some of my loneliest times. I developed an eating disorder, starving myself until I felt weak and frequently dizzy. At the time, I believed this was about body image. Simple aesthetics. Now I think it was a form of self-harm and a cry for help – an attempt to give my invisible internal misery a physical manifestation, that would be visible on the outside. I imagined some angelic all-knowing being who would do what needed to be done, to fix me. It was noticed by some. My

Mum showed concern and asked me what it was about. I gave her the body image spiel that I still believed myself (and which was part of the truth). She asked my father (a doctor) for advice. He suggested having my iron levels tested for anaemia but said he wasn't concerned because I was still menstruating, and he was sure I wouldn't keep it up too long as I loved food too much. To be clear, I know these people were trying to help me in the ways they knew how and I always knew I was loved.

In the end, what saved me physically was an unplanned pregnancy. I could justify using my body against myself but not putting my baby in harm's way. I don't know what would have happened if I continued my hunger strike. My daughter may have saved my life.

I had three children, each pregnancy followed by a descent into post-natal depression. After my first pregnancy, I told my general practitioner (GP) that I was feeling run down. I didn't really recognise the depression. I was a sleep-deprived single mother. Of course, I felt run down! My doctor told me he thought I was a bit depressed and prescribed daily walks with the pram. After my second pregnancy, I was again convinced the torturous lack of sleep was my real problem, but I remember frightening thoughts and a horrible flatness that wouldn't shift. During this time friends from overseas came to stay and I found myself barely able to speak to them. I was plodding through those days knowing my behaviour wasn't right, but unable to muster any strength to even pretend. Sometimes I was just sitting awkwardly with them, blank faced and speechless, but painfully aware of the awfulness of it all.

After the traumatic delivery of my third baby the depression returned in force and I became gripped by an overwhelming, panicky worry about the future of the planet. With the effects of climate change constantly in the media and noticeably all around me, I felt like I was living in the final days of the earth. It was a crushing sense of impending doom riddled with the guilt of inflicting living – through these final days – on my newborn baby and children. What was I thinking bringing them into a world where they had no future? I had visions of tripping down the stairs and cracking my head on concrete, collisions with semi-trailers or even better, a brain tumour which would enable me to leave the world quietly in a hospital bed with the comfort of pain medications. Deaths that wouldn't leave my family with the pain of knowing I wanted it.

I was referred to a child and family health counsellor. On my first visit with her, as I was trying to explain my feelings, I remember saying "I'm not sure if I'm actually depressed". She answered "well, let me answer that one for you, there's no question you are". This was a turning point for me. Here was someone who saw me and heard me and validated my experience and emotions. She walked with me through the next two years, through starting medication, trialing and changing drugs and doses. There were times I felt completely hopeless, and there were easier times. She told me "I'm in until you give me the sack". For as long as I needed her she was committed to be there.

I never told her how close I came to suicide. How one day, I was convinced my usual logic was wrong and my family would be better off without me. That now was the best time because my children were young enough not to remember me. I drove away from home alone under the guise of going to the shops, completely certain I wouldn't go back. I have no memory of how I ended up safely back at home. I do know that counsellor saved my life.

It hasn't been smooth sailing since then. I have had several more episodes of major depression, times feeling completely hopeless, with the most soul crushing feelings of despair. Many of us are familiar with the analogy of depression as a black dog. I see my depression as a bird. In the best times it's a peaceful black cockatoo, flapping quietly high in the sky. Or a little blackbird that perches on my head. It opens it beak and sings to the sky. On bleaker days, a sinister black crow digs its claws into my shoulder and caws loudly in my ear. That sharp beak hovering in my peripheral vision poised to attack. And sometimes my depression is a monstrous raven. Towering over me, it envelops me in its wings. I am cast into complete darkness. Warmth, happiness, comfort and hope vanish along with the light.

Accepting my depression and anxiety as familiar parts of my life that will never leave me – helps completely. It brings a sense of walking alongside myself and recognising what state I am currently in. Sometimes I can even acknowledge the gifts the birds have brought me: empathy, compassion, strength and resilience, gifts of self-awareness and courage.

I have been getting a lot more help: counselling, pain specialists for my chronic pain, a psychiatrist to review my medications and an empathic GP. As more walls around the topic of mental health come down, I feel less alone. I hear others voicing their experiences. A blogger I have read for a long time, firstly for her crafty posts, and then more for her wonderfully practical tips for dealing with tough times, has been particularly inspiring. She is an expert at self-care. An expert at acknowledging her feelings and being conscious of small things that make living through the bad times more comfortable – not in an abstract way, but by concrete acts of compassion towards herself. I have learned that cocooning myself in a blanket on a comfy chair with my favourite tea and hand stitching or knitting something (or nothing) is cosy and soothing and quietly eases me back towards myself. I know when the best thing I can do is take to my bed and allow myself to sleep. I now see these small acts of kindness towards myself as highly productive rather than a failure to function in the ways I should. I am learning to be braver and to shed the victim skin I have worn. I can usually remember to also forgive myself for the times I don't manage things well. I am so grateful for the kind of sharing which helps me learn these precious things.

I know that there will be more days when I am smothered by black wings. I will not be able to believe it will ever pass or remember feeling better. There will be more days when I long to fall asleep and never wake up. Nothing will feel like a gift. On another day, I probably couldn't write with any hope or positivity but today I can think bravely, that what is coming will come, and I will meet it when it does. Today I welcome the blackbird whose weight is light on my head. Its face is lifted to the sky. I'm listening to hear it sing.

Kylie would love to see a kinder experience for people living with invisible difficulties, mental or otherwise. She feels strongly about promoting compassion, empathy and kindness and working to break down the stigma and judgement silently felt by so many. Kylie finds solace in nature and creativity.

The Anxiety Template
Mark Thompson

Newton's third law states that everything must have an equal and opposite reaction. I would argue that most things have an unequal and opposite over-reaction.

But then, I have a chronic anxiety issue.

I haven't studied it or written papers on it like Newton, but I have and do live with it. It's a daily companion. Every word, every conversation, every decision analysed, taken outside and beaten severely with a cricket bat until it's too exhausted to pick a side. The wholeness of time will make the decision for me, and opportunities will fly by whilst my body and mind fight amongst themselves trying to assess danger and risk.

Apple or orange?

Simple question but it can trigger virtual office assistants on either shoulder to compete with louder and increasingly aggressive arguments trying to pull me to their side – logical vs emotional. What's safe? What's not? What have I seen? What haven't I? It's automatic... "Hey, it looks like you're writing a letter! Which anxiety formatting would you like to use? Cry? Stress? Aggression? Run away?"

I don't think physical symptoms of anxiety necessarily need to be explained, but often anxiety and panic attacks can look different depending on the individual. And this is where the anxiety formatting comes in – much like a bad Office template, mine may seem like a textbook obvious anxiety template to others but to me, each whirlwind, each vortex feels like a real threat – a real chance to unearth the catastrophe that will make sure 'the bad thing' happens.

Will my good-natured jape cause untold damage to this person? What does this oddly placed blue sticker come to mean in my life and should I take notice of it? Did that person just insult me, and I don't understand because I'm too stupid? What if I replied wrong to that email back in 2007 and it's only just been found, and now someone will ring me tomorrow and bring it up? Do I want a cup of tea that a colleague just innocently offered?

Any of these can bring up anxiety office assistant. And I'd like to claim that this is where decisions are made but in reality, the assistant takes over and quickly promotes itself to anxiety office dictator. The fight / flight / freeze response manages to happen all at the same time and it's a virtual poker machine of responses scrolling behind my eyes that lead to an internal conflict that's barely recognisable from anything that I'd be able to adequately describe.

Run! Stay! Ask for clarification! Just do something! ANYTHING!

Part of me would love to know what I look like when I'm in this place but part of me hates the idea. I spend so long here that I'm convinced that 'Virtual poker machine' should adequately describe my 'look' and I think it would be a great addition to this year's spring and summer anxiety fashion catalogue. Mainly so that I can recognise my people...

The constantness of anxiety makes life tiring. The only defence and fight back I realistically have is humour. There has to be a point to this. An upside. A light at the end of the tunnel. A bonus point that balances out the unfairness of needing constant reassurance that anxiety dictator has a little clickable red 'x' in the top right hand corner. Those who love me provide this, often unconditionally. It's reassuring and without it, I can get lost quickly.

It goes further too. I think of events from my past that could've created the sliding doors moments: the day I started carrying a knife, the head banging on a solid window, the screaming and holding my head to keep it all inside there, the threat in the street, the car at the bus stop.

And these moments inevitably lead to well-intentioned, but ill-conceived, advice from professionals and non-professionals alike:

"Just breathe!"
"We ALL suffer from anxiety, it can be normal!"
"You'd be better if you took your meds!"

In certain circumstances, it's all solid advice but when something else is at the wheel it's difficult to make those decisions. Equally, anxiety leaves me with an overwhelming sense of needing to control the environment – the dictated to becoming the dictator – and so I need to be able to ask people around me to support me.

It's easy to write, it's hard to do. "Just ask for help!" is a good message but practically, how easy is it to get that support? In my case, I'm lucky. I have people who can, will and do support me. They create safety for me to try things and throughout the years I have progressed from housebound agoraphobic, to productive member of society with goals, dreams, achievements and further aspirations – holding hands with deep seated insecurities and anxiety assistants of varying levels of aggression, a constant and unfriendly passenger.

That's the thing, office dictator doesn't always allow me to be me. If I need a situation to change I need it to change, and I can't always put my mind into the right space to communicate in the way I know I can. I'm fortunate that most people in my life allow for this, and what can come across as controlling to others, is often sickening anxiety, panic and stress about what is going to come next – what if, what if, what if?

The added level of emotional toil this takes on the soul can be damaging. But on the other side of the coin, my appreciation jug fills to the brim with relatively mundane occurrences which others may see as inconvenience.

My car radio does not work when the weather is hot, but the opportunity to be frustrated on a drive home from work by a minor inconvenience is a joy to someone who once considered three steps into the back yard in the dark as an achievement.

I can't claim to know how to fix chronic anxiety, how to stop the difficulty of it from turning into a dark depressive episode or worse. I can't say how others should go about attacking it. From what I know, each person has a unique relationship with their own anxieties and they come from different experiences.

In my job I regularly get asked how it all changed. "What did **you** do? How did **you** become 'better'?" The answer to this question is impossible to sum up in just a few words. Primarily connection to people whilst anchoring myself to interests which keep me interacting with the world.

It was a decision. It was definitely a decision. I didn't know what recovery was. But I knew that advice to go for a walk every day or to alter my sleep routine or to breathe or try these meds didn't sit well. I did those steps of course, but it felt empty.

And this is when I actively chose to engage in recovery – recovery had to have a point, recovery had to have meaning, I had to contribute. If I was going to be well and be part of anything resembling the real world I had to do what 'real people' did. I now understand that I was merely going by the markers that others set down as contributing. But it created connection.

I somehow managed to volunteer – and on day one I called back after hours, to check whether I had stuck stamps on envelopes correctly such was my fear of failure and being wrong. And obviously, of making the call itself!

Ultimately this led to many other pathways opening up – some taken, some missed – but it taught me that I could contribute whilst being overwhelmed, in spite of fear, in spite of internal conflict. It led me to a place of being able to say "yes", despite the fears of the world ending, of never-ending shame, despite the nagging questions and self-doubt. Learning to be active whilst internally suffering was a game changer.

It's not *quite* as simple as just making a decision – it took a long time to reach that place. Recovery for me was and continues to be about contributing and purpose. Throw in awareness, strategies and connection but primarily I find that having reasons to do things is what keeps invading thoughts at bay.

And a certain amount of acceptance. Whilst I can try to add new perspectives, try new things and find new strategies there is a certain comfort in knowing that, regardless of what the waves bring, I can still offer something. There's value there and the world is different for my presence in it.

I am a dedicated peer worker, creative worrier and leaving things until the last minute ninja. I appreciate and embrace my struggles and big feelings. They make me appreciate my comfortable couch. In real life I watch much sport, take many photos and play too many computer games. I am also an optimist. Whatever it is, you can do it.

A Madful Life – 3 Random Acts
Jude D.

Act 1 – A fragmented start

Abused yet hardly touched
Destroyed by secrets hushed,
Silence far deadlier than any spoken word
Inferences drawn from the silence heard.

Alone, too little to understand,
As others bury their heads in sand
Protector? Abuser? Or just neglect?
Inside our head, trapped emotions collect.

Thoughts racing round and round and round,
Screaming out, but without a sound
No way to escape or leave this place,
But inside our head that is not the case.

Leave it to someone older, stronger
Parts who can cope for longer,
For in our head, fantasy was true
And love and affection were things that we knew.

Act 2 – *The Challenges of Opportunity: My NDIS experience**

I don't want to be told I'm eligible then hear *nothing* for forty weeks,
Nor information sessions so confusing and rushed I can't understand the
woman who speaks.

I don't want to be told we can't get the rollout right due to its massive
scale,
From people who don't comprehend the impact of *every single* fail.
I don't want to be stigmatised by being labelled, 'permanently' disabled,
I want help and support so my life can be stable.
I'm tired of constantly being promised 'choice' and 'control',
When more often than not, I feel trapped in a big… black… hole.
For me, this system is not just an optional extra,
Some nice idea written on butchers' paper with Texta.
I need support to function, to thrive…
But I also need help just to stay alive!
I'm sick of the guilt I feel for the demands placed on my 'informal carer',
I crave a world that's gentler and fairer.
I don't need more bureaucracy, buck-passing and paperwork,
I'm sick of decisions that are incongruent, reactions knee-jerk.
Some things in life can't be compressed into simple goals,
Written on plans, full of conditions; agreements full of loop-holes.
Maybe I'm remiss to crave certainty in an uncertain world,
But my head is full of dreams, yet all jumbled and swirled.
My psych says I'm discombobulated, over-sensitive, and I'm often unsafe,
And this whole NDIS process, it is starting to chafe.
You promise me a future full of capacity and hope,
Yet fail to recognise, that right NOW, I… just… can't… cope.
For years I've lost workers and groups (and friends) I still grieve,
From a system that's callous, heart-less or perhaps just naïve.
You read the reports but do you *understand* the words?
The desperation, the fear, the loneliness – it all seems unheard.
I'm not really sure I have the strength to endure
A process this haphazard, fragmented and unsure.

Some days I just want it all to go away,
The distress and frustration seem to outweigh…
The offer of an *ordinary* life – of my choosing,
It really all seems rather insane and bemusing.
But what can I do, trapped in limbo, descending
To a point where I contemplate it all… just ending?
The ideals of connection, meaning and opportunity,
Of finally feeling a real part of my community
Dangle in front like a carrot just out of reach
Whilst the pain in my heart continues to screech.
But no-one's listening and no-one hears
The disabling distress, the silent tears.
So, I struggle along, one foot in front of the other,
As governments make one change after another.
I hope and I pray for the strength to go on,
Please may this NDIS-thing not all be one big con.
For with the right supports, at just the right time,
Who knows to what heights, I just might climb?

Yet I know even then I shan't relax,
For there are so many others falling through the cracks.
A system set up for the most vulnerable and exposed,
With so few safety-nets considered or proposed?
Our society needs to be better than this,
No more excuses and things all amiss.
For everyone, especially those of us who struggle,
Those of us for whom our lives are a complete muddle,
Deserve dignity and care – the most basic right
And for this we must ALL continue the fight!

---

* *The NDIS is Australia's National Disability Insurance Scheme – the main way that community-based psycho-social disability supports are currently being delivered in Victoria.*

Act 3 – What if...?

What if I accept that maybe, just maybe, I am good enough
What if I can have inner gentleness, but still be tough
What if I decide, despite the odds, there is a way
What if I believed, I am okay
What if I can learn that love needn't be feared
What if I can still see through my eyes all teared
What if I realised that life is to live, not just endure
What if I stopped looking for that elusive cure
What if I embraced my madness in all its glory
What if I learned when, and how, to best tell my story
What if I slowed right down, slower still...
What if I reimagine the dreams that I can never fulfil
What if I could navigate my own connections
What if I could handle the pain of rejections
What if I could let past hurts just go
What if their lessons retained wisdom I'd know
What if I, myself, defined my peers
What if mutual support could last for years
What if it was okay to talk of death
What if I understood the value of *every* breath
What if roller coasters could be fun, not just metaphor
What if self-compassion was fundamental to my core
What if I could become indifferent to those who've harmed me
What if I could access those things that calmed me
What if I could see the colour amongst all the grey,
And what if, what if, I could start all of this today?

Jude D lives in Melbourne, thinks she's lazy but actually does too much and is completely delusional about how many hours there are in each day; some days she can't leave the house, other days she thinks she can change the world. She is passionate about her family and friends (especially her five gorgeous nephews and dog), lived experience/mental health/ community advocacy and enjoys live theatre and watching TV (with veggie pizza and ice-cream.)

Unbecoming
Katie Shead

When you hear the terms 'mental distress' or 'extreme state' you tend to think of states of high emotion; thoughts race 100 miles an hour, shaking, overwhelming mental pain. But extremes have two ends and every extreme emotional high that the mind is capable of is balanced, somewhere, by an extreme emotional low: numbness, disconnection from the world around you, and unbecoming.

I have Dissociative Identity Disorder (DID) and as part of it I experience something probably most correctly termed 'dissociative catatonia'. However, I prefer to describe it as 'unbecoming', it makes it sound less clinical and, to be honest, I think it's a more accurate description.

Technically, it's an advantageous learned response. If you are in a traumatic situation and you have no ability to fight and no ability to run away then the next best thing is to let your mind escape when your body can't. This is dissociation. Like many other things dissociation exists on a spectrum. At one end you have daydreaming, a brief, harmless disconnection from reality that can end at any time; at the other end you have DID, in which your very self fractures in order to help you cope with a trauma you cannot escape. Within this fracturing I have found a further dissociation, one originally intended to help me escape when even the fracturing of my self was not enough to protect me. In this state, what is left of me unravels leaving nothing behind that could be hurt.

Unfortunately this ability, once learned, can't really be switched off, and once the original need for it is past, it does not fade into nothingness.

Instead, dissociative catatonia is now a part of my everyday life, just as much as sleeping or breathing.

To someone looking at me during this type of episode I seem like I could almost be asleep; my body sits motionless, except for my eyes which are open and blinking, but unseeing. You can speak to me, but I won't respond. Wave a hand in front of my face and the most you'll get is another blink. Sometimes, when it gets bad enough, you can touch my arm, hold my hand, even pick me up, and I'll give no indication that I've felt anything.

I know I described emotional highs and lows as being opposite extremes, but for me they lead into each other. When I am overwhelmed I feel it building, my thoughts are racing, jumping from one half-formed thing to the next so fast that I cannot keep up. The world feels like it's closing in, and my mind is receiving so many different types of information so quickly that it feels like it is going to burst open.

It keeps building, higher and higher.

And then it stops.

Everything melts away. I feel my muscles unclench and the thoughts drain out of my head. I'm not shaking anymore and my hands lie limp in my lap. I don't feel anything anymore, I'm beyond the point where emotion can fill me up like an over-blown balloon. I can no longer hear the sound of someone fidgeting metres away from me, in fact, I can't hear someone talking while sitting next to me. It's like a thick wall has gone up between me and the rest of the world. It blocks everything out. It protects me.

It protects me?

The initial relief is one of the most wonderful feelings, like cool water on a 40 degree day, but it doesn't stop once the panic, pain, and agitation have left. Once my hands have stopped shaking I then start to feel the numbness spread from the tips of my fingers, up along my arms. It spreads up my arms, up my legs and across my cheekbones, a slow petrification that pulls me out of my own body. I can look at my hands and they look like the hands of a stranger. I've never seen them before. They can't be mine. They don't move when I ask them to. Have I ever had hands?

I never knew that nothing could be such a strong feeling.

Even as I sit here writing this, I feel phantom numbness in my hands and then spreading down my arms. It hasn't gone further than my elbows and I can still type, but they feel like they belong to someone else. I'm remotely piloting fingers that don't belong to me. But it's okay. I still know who I am and I know that eventually I will be able to look down and see where my hands attach to my forearms and forearms reach my elbow, but for now I will just keep writing. My fingers might not be my own, but while they can still press the keys words can travel from my mind to the page.

When I have a full episode I don't know any of that, my thoughts flow out of my mind as the life flows out of my limbs. Soon I am alone. My mind is encased in a vacuum, nothing can reach me and I can't reach out, not because I'm unable, but because there's not enough thought left in me to want anything.

And then, inside that vacuum, I start to flow away as well. My self unravels, like an old jumper coming apart stitch by stitch. My mind becomes a foreign country I've never been to.

I'm unbecoming

I'm unbecome

I'm un

I'm

I

...

Whatever I am, it is outside time. It is everything, but at the same time it is nothing at all. I both am and am not, if there's even enough left to be either. Time passes, or maybe it just jumps and suddenly it is Later.

When Later arrives my mind trickles back, knitting together stitch by stitch. I begin to hear voices moving around me. Soon I begin to recognise them, the words have meanings again and the thoughts slink back into my head, but my mind is still too weighed down to catch them. So I wait.

I wait, frozen, until sounds become words and words become meaning and meaning becomes understanding.

After Later I begin to realise that I can see flashes of colour. They swirl about in meaningless patterns before my mind can catch up and decode what it means when these colours sit next to each other. Slowly I begin to find the meaning of these colours and shapes, and the world pieces together in front of my eyes. One by one the shapes come into focus – blurred flashes become faces, swirls become hair, and swathes of colour become walls.

Later I *am*, after Later the world *is*.

Once we both *are* the heaviness begins to slip from my fingers and after a Time my body *is* too. It slips back on like warm pyjamas and I know it's mine.

I'm home.

I will continue to unbecome and become for the rest of my life. Some days I am only half of me, others the world feels like a dream I don't recognise. This isn't something that can be cured, only managed and it has been with me for as long as I can remember. It can be terrifying to come back to reality with no idea what has happened to you. In these situations my body is entirely vulnerable. Anything could happen to me and I might never know. It is the price my mind pays in order to keep itself safe, because sometimes not knowing is better.

There are some things that I try to do to relieve the fear of slipping quietly away and losing myself forever, drifting in limbo and unable to knit myself back together again. The relief of being able to slip away into nothing as an escape can become comforting after a time and I try to focus on it when I start to drown in the hopelessness that comes alongside a chronic condition. It helps a bit, not a lot, but that's what DID is like for me, finding ways to offset small bits of distress and sitting through what cannot be changed, waiting until I'm me again, and then preparing for the next time I unbecome.

I was diagnosed with Dissociative Identity Disorder when I was 18, but it probably emerged when I was 6-7. Our system has 11 members and we do our best to work together for the good of the whole. In my everyday life I research archaeology because I like exploring the mindsets of ancient peoples and understanding what motivated them.

ANIMA KILLS ME
Oliver Damian

She often comes to me unawares. Some mornings I feel her as I wake up with this feeling of a debilitating heaviness weighing on my body. She comes with a sense of tiredness that no amount of rest or sleep could ever abate. She shotguns me with pellets of doubt. What's the point of it all? I'm in my bedroom all alone. Like yesterday. Like last year. Like five years ago. Like forever. If I die now, how long will it take before anyone notices that I'm gone? I get images of me hanging myself. The rope around my neck hanging over the balcony. By the doorway. From the rooftop. A dramatic jump from the 21st floor will do it. How about the sharpest kitchen knife slashing flawlessly over my throat. The blood splatter creating a Rorschach Test that will keep future forensic psychologists entertained forever. Poison? There's plenty under the kitchen sink and under the bathroom vanity kit. Maybe kill my flatmate, my neighbours first. How about the whole world? Destroy the whole universe? Collapse the multiverses? Make time stop. Run backwards. Let everything that is good and beautiful turn dark and ugly.

Her voice feels like a billion thorns stabbing at my confused heart. I'm forced to flee the burned houses, the shallow graves, and the anguished faces of the past. Yet time and again I run towards the warmth of her body as it wakes from the night's sleep. I have this fantasy of staying forever in her primordial embrace. I long for the undulating comfort of her breasts. The smooth plains of her skin. But deep in me, I know this is a paper thin dream. Stretched in a distended horizon, her pashmina of comfort gets burned by the sniggering of the morning sun.

Her water blue eyes reach out to the almost wet sky and the red shimmering earth. The oven-dry wind makes watery waves of her streaky blonde hair. It bakes her porcelain skin reddish pink. A million years behind her, from that almost forgotten galaxy, I see the shadow of a man. He is still bombarding her with radio waves that melt the sweet fairy floss on her curious tongue. An older woman is still somewhere out there. She helps her grow wings, coax her horns out, pull her tail out, time and again from the days of cuddly teddy bears to last week's killer stilettos. They're all hiding in a closet of secrets and dreams.

In the basement, there is a frothy rich cocktail of airline tickets, postcards, and bus rides. A band of androgynous youth plays psychedelic tunes to lead a horde of nymph-etic desires into a sea of bucolic sirens, and fairies. The incubus prey-fully waits in the darkest nooks and crannies of the sea cave night.

Inside I am more frozen than Antartica, more barren than the Nullabor.

Oh how much I want to kiss and bite the moon's shining face. Let dirty blood stain her proud immaculate glow. Hey, moon! Stop pulling at the substances of my inner being. I give up. I surrender. I cannot rise from the earth and meet you up there where you will never come down.

I feel ice all around me. My arms are frozen. My stomach is grumbling. I feel soot. I smell the stench. Behind the heavy wooden door, I hear laughter. I smell food. I imagine love. Yet I remain outside. Dying of cold. I feel eyes around me thumbing their noses with disgust. I whisper "Mummy please hold me tight, where are you?". A white-hot knife plunges into my heart that melts like butter. I sink into this quicksand of filth. Voices cry out for help. Everywhere death and rotting flesh. A vice grip of darkness clamps me in. I hear a voice. I follow it. I stand firm. I look at your eyes. I hold the gaze. I feel the mists lift. I feel tickling in my tummy. I feel the pleasure of fire gushing in from below.

Wheezing. Wooozzzing. Wobbling. Winging. I feel like lava lamp liquid. Bobbing up, down, left, right, all around. I swirl in this milky moon froth of ecstasy. I feel you in me. I feel me in you. We feel you. I, him, her, us, and them. No, not me. Not you. Not them. Not us. Only be. Zipping. Zwoooshing. Zwonking. Zapping. Time bends. Backwards, forwards, sideways. Here, today, yesterday, tomorrow, never, before, always.

Untangling the knots of no, never, not there. I swiftly glide in this molten sea of wanting. Continents shift with the sheer breath of her eyes. She claws through the black-velvet night of my soul. This little man must die if I am to fly with the feral freedom of her fire.

I feel this giant knot in my heart. The sins of the father slither with the abandonment of the mother. The pussy little boy rears its big ugly head. His paper-thin personality crumpled and torn. Tossed from bin to bin. He feels mute, deaf, numb. His eyes feel dry. But tonight he can feel. He can cry. In the darkness of the night, he can feel a little joey tucked inside the pouch of his fragility.

I feel the sweet taste of her freedom like wild horses galloping to the sea. I fear yet I'm most fascinated by her. I can do nothing but slowly meander through the mists of her mysteries. Gently drenched by her presence I can't help but love.

Oliver was raised by his paternal grandparents in a tiny village in the Philippines. His father who was an accountant was the first person in the village to get a university degree. His mother was a young Vietnamese accountant on secondment to Manila who promptly went back to Saigon after Oliver was born. Oliver was 13 when he first met her. Needless to say these events had deep reverberations in his life.
http://www.oliver-damian.space

Healing relationships
Stephanie Mitchell

When I think of my healing journey the most striking thing that stands out to me is the numerous people who have offered me love, hope and acceptance as I fumbled my way through the ups and downs of my experience. There are other important moments, like finding meaningful work and seeking out an integrative GP who helped me sort out some epigenetic problems that were making it very hard for me to think clearly, but the most life changing experiences have always happened in relationships.

To paraphrase Carl Jung: the wounds that were created in relationship can only be healed in relationship[1]. This has been the largest part of my experience. It was like I really couldn't find myself by myself. I needed people who could see me as different to how I saw myself, so I could begin to consider myself differently. This has been the key to unlocking my inner torment.

My childhood had been a terrifying time where I tried to find some place of safety in a chaotic and violent environment. This is not to say that it was bereft of moments of kindness or care, but I walked through my days with a pervasive sense of danger and this over-rode most of my other experiences.

I was also fed a steady diet of being 'too, something'. It didn't seem to matter what I did it was wrong. Too loud, too needy, too naughty, too stupid, too much... and always the violence.

---

1 *Carl Jung (1875-1961) Swiss psychiatrist and psychoanalyst.*

During this time my mother let me know that what was going on in our home wasn't right, and so I grew up searching for this 'right' thing that was lacking in our family. While my mother was often stretched and unable to be there for me or see me, she did offer me the gift of perspective and from about the age of eight I went in search of what a 'right' family looked like. I spent countless hours visiting new mums in our street and taking mental notes about how this different thing was done. I found out that to be nurtured is something a child needs and deserves and I began to consider what my life might be like if I had this.

I moved into my adult life quite determined that I would have a different experience from my family of origin. I didn't know how this would happen, but I was sure I was not going to replicate the train wreck that was my parents' relationship by staying with someone who didn't adore me whole heartedly… even if I was 'too something'. I had a naïve fantasy that I might grow up and find a person to love me and make it all better. Somehow, I found the person who would love me for all my intensity and brokenness, however this didn't produce the 'happily ever after' that I had hoped for. I still carried terrible inner scars from all abuse I had suffered, and it felt like I was possessed by something that just knew I was a vile and worthless creature, and more importantly, that the world was a very very scary place.

I moved through the next 20 years of my life trying to keep away from this scary world as much as I could.

I home-schooled my children and it was during this time that I met a group of home-schooling mums who embraced and loved me, and I began to feel some small sense of safety in the world. Being soaked in the acceptance of this community I had a striking experience that gave me pause to re-consider some of the things I believed about myself. A good friend and fellow home-schooling parent, Debbie, said to me "Stephanie, your intensity and vulnerability is a gift to everyone around you". I was deeply touched by this comment and also completely shocked. Someone inside my head was yelling "What the hell? What planet does she live on?!" I wanted to push her away and keep all that crazy talk a long way away from me. A part of me knew that if I let myself believe it was ok to be as intense or angry or needy as I felt inside, that this thing that I kept hidden would come rushing out and overtake me, and nobody would be celebrating that! This encounter stuck in my head and even though I couldn't yet accept it, I would hold onto this moment and these words for many, many years.

Once my children were finished with their schooling, I returned to work as a Peer Worker. I was thoroughly attached to my identity of being broken, so this role seemed to be the right place for me to begin to venture back into the big, scary, world. In this role I was fortunate to meet a mental health nurse named Matt Ball. We were both reading Mad in America and listening to Madness Radio and we struck up a friendship over our passion to change the mental health system. His belief in me as 'not broken' was incomprehensible to me. Here was an incredibly talented and intelligent person working at the cutting edge of mental health who told me that I had something to offer. The cogs in my head began to turn once more.

At this time my employer offered for me to train as a counsellor and in a moment of what seemed like sheer stupidity and arrogance, I applied for the course, knowing I may never complete it.

Shortly after this my life took an unexpected turn and I was triggered into a frightening and dark place that I feared I might never return from. I was thoroughly suicidal and utterly utterly terrified. There seemed to be no end to this dark place, and I felt myself flailing in an abyss where I couldn't gain a hold of anything to steady myself. Every facet of life seemed to contain some danger and I became increasingly paranoid of the things that would come after me and also surely others. As I slowly found my way out of this state (that I like to call a 'PTSD crisis') I realised that I had just faced one of my biggest fears. I was messy beyond belief and my husband and those closest to me hadn't once said I was "too anything". In fact, shortly after this I was invited to apply for a job at an NGO where I had been co-facilitating a voice hearers' group.

I was incredulous. Only a few months earlier I had been attended the group in a state of terror, shaking and rambling about my fears, and now they wanted to offer me a job? I secured the job and my life turned in a new direction, as I found myself again in relationships where people believed in me.

During this time, I decided I needed to go back into therapy. I have had a lot of therapy in the past but none of this previous work made a difference to how I felt inside my skin. I felt that I was constantly trying to use my mind to manage my internal experience and it was exhausting. I wanted something different. I had to believe that there was hope that I wouldn't always be tormented by the pervasive fear that raged inside me. I pushed back against DBT (Dialectical Behaviour Therapy) and ACT (Acceptance Commitment Therapy) and other cognitive based approaches, and even the 'Recovery' movement that told me the best I could expect was to live well with what I was given and build up my 'skills' to be more resilient.

No! I wanted healing, damn it!

During one of those everyday conversations you have with colleagues when you work in a therapeutic service, my good friend and mentor, Ben Swift, mentioned Internal Family Systems Therapy (IFS) to me. I was looking to undertake some more trauma therapy training and he thought this would be a good place to start. As I began looking into IFS it made a lot of sense to me in the context of my own trauma and so I decided to give it a try. I had no idea when I signed up, that my life was about to completely change. I found an IFS therapist, who offered a space of safety to be with the parts of myself that had been so hidden in darkness for so long. I was finally able to process my trauma history in a safe way and help the parts of myself that have been so vilified, to find healing and a new perspective on life and myself.

I am still in therapy at the point of writing this chapter, but my internal experience has shifted significantly. The most striking change is that I don't feel afraid all the time.

It seems to me that only through the journey of acceptance in relationship was I able to find a truly healing relationship with my own inner experience, and a difference sense of who I am from the inside out.

Stephanie is a psychotherapist who specializes in working with complex trauma from an Internal Family Systems perspective. Stephanie has extensive experience facilitating therapeutic groups and is interested in how healing occurs in the space of human connection. Stephanie has a passion for working with people experiencing things that are often labelled extreme or unusual, including those diagnosed with BPD and schizophrenia. Stephanie works in private practice as Co-Director of the HUMANE Clinic Adelaide. (www.humaneclinic.com.au)

Connection: Knowing like Breathing
Jenny Hickinbotham

For nearly sixty years I have had problems connecting.

What is connection? Various forms of human connection include:

Spoken connection or conversation between two or more people.

Spoken inner, mental connection between two or more people.

Touch

Feel

Gesture

Smell

Much more

Connection for me was fractured, from a very young age. People hurt and abused me, physically, sexually, emotionally, psychologically, spiritually. I did not want to connect with anyone, except the dog. I wanted to be in my own, private space. I wanted to be left alone. I would have been happiest dead, or at least, not alive on this earth.

What did this mean in my daily life?

My mother forced me to leave the house to attend duties, which always resulted in connection with other people. She forced me to speak (connect) to neighbours... she forced me to go to the grocer (connect) ... she forced me to go to school (multiple connections) ... she forced me to church (multiple connections) ... at family gatherings, social or community events, I was forced to connect with others and unfortunately, often to KISS.

The form of connection I hated most, was internal voices, people connecting psychologically. For me, the learned feeling and sense of powerlessness was palpable, bodily. However, it's important to acknowledge, that people do connect psychologically without hurting or abusing each other, it's a normal human experience. Some people do it unconsciously, others do it consciously.

As I grew my identity became fragmented and questionable. Who was I? I thought I was to blame for the way I was, the isolation I sought, the way people had, and on occasion still did, engage inappropriately with me, took advantage, abused me. It was my own fault. I brought it on myself. It was because I was bad, unlovable. The shame, guilt and blame were unbearable.

I had two brothers, and a father, which forced me to consider the male population in a different light, I still struggled. At primary school, I always had one friend. However, my relationship with my mother was difficult, she pushed me to function 'normally'. She stole my friends. Now that I am much older, I can see that she had identity fractures too. She was lonely. Mother wanted me to be her friend, she always told me that her mother was her best friend. My relationship with my mother was challenged, since she had abandoned me to our town bank manager and his wife, when I was six-years-old. She travelled overseas to join my father for three months. I was chronically abused, and when she came home I did not recognize her. She never believed my stories, not then and not later. My love for her was grossly challenged and I found our relationship difficult. As she could not have me as a friend, she stole my friends.

I managed to survive my teenage years, because I went to an all-girls school. My results were terrible, I looked at some old reports just a few weeks ago, I got Es, Ds, and occasionally Cs. I did make a few girlfriends. I remember going on a sleep-over, what an atrocious mistake. I accused the father of the family of being a pedophile, using my internal voice, of course, I couldn't speak the words out loud. He was, understandably, very defensive and upset, which played out in strained connections, my physical reluctance to go anywhere near the man. I never went outside our family home for extended periods again, until a tennis camp was recommended. During high school, I played tennis every weekend and I loved it, although, I was never a killer player.

My parents talked me into going to the tennis camp. I was super, super, anxious and panicky. I packed my tennis clothes, I hated that my dresses were so short, but I had my racket. I got on a bus, but I can't remember where we traveled, I was dissociating. I remember playing tennis, a lot of tennis and I have a vague concept of acknowledging, "oh, those people are not so bad".

I went overseas, to California, to attend high school. My older brother had gone to Bordeaux in France when he was in year 11, so I insisted on the equal opportunity. Again, I was anxious, but all went well. I wanted to get away from my mother's voice. She'd had a break-down when I was about fourteen, now she talked constantly in my head. The two older siblings of the Californian family I lived with were very kind. Philip took me backpacking to Yosemite Mountains and Betty got me a job babysitting her boyfriend's three much younger brothers. At high-school I studied psychology and Patricia, the teacher, became a voice in my head helping me with my mother voice/relationship, although I knew Patricia was a voice in my head, I didn't really acknowledge her consciously.

Back in Melbourne I started at Teachers College but dropped out within a couple of years. I couldn't handle the practical sessions, where children who had differences were ignored, shunned, abandoned by the teacher and other children, they were isolated, made to feel like freaks. I drifted from job to job.

Connection, is everything. Do you feel a psychological connection with the people you love? Or are you only connected when physically associated?

I started to hear difficult voices only a few years later. I moved to Adelaide to get away from my family, all the time I was trying to get help, like Patricia. I knew I had experienced trauma, but these memories were unreachable fragments. Finally, I met a social worker who agreed to become the voice in my head. I began to recall my difficult childhood. Shame, blame and guilt were extremely destructive experiences as I experienced memories, flashbacks and nightmares. The dominant voice I heard insisted that I was to blame for all that had happened to me. I was totally gutted, sad and self-destructive.

My illness became so acute I moved back to Melbourne for support. My survival strategies included taking on other identities. If I heard the inner voice, I would pretend to be someone else, in both my body and mind. Over time, I developed various recurring identities, such as my dead brother, which I applied when trying to escape the voice. The voice wanted to know what I was doing, so I provided a continuous running commentary, inside my head, where I was, what I was doing, who I was with, my plans. Another escape strategy was to read everything I saw, signs, marketing, number plates, reading aloud inside my head. I hated being in public, I would stare at a corner of the room, draw lines and patterns with my perceptions, and dissociate. I did negative self-talk, many people do, it is a learned form of self-abuse.

Skip forward thirty years. I now know that main voice, the one refusing to take responsibility, trying to blame me, was my mother. Further, I had recently recalled she abused me in a once off event too. She did everything she could, using both external and internal voices, to stop me recalling and acknowledging her abuse. She denied any responsibility for my torture by other people from our town.

I was always convinced of the reality of the voices I heard inside my head. After Patricia, I briefly saw Ayleen in 1987, who asked me if the voices came from within my head or from an outside source. I thought this was a trick question, if I answered wrong, I would be put into a strait jacket and incarcerated in a mental institution. I said my voices originated from outside my body. She just nodded. Returning from Adelaide to Melbourne, I went to CASA and was referred to their Freudian psychiatrist, he told me the voice I heard was my mother's. I left that guy, no doubt, my 'voice', my mother, giving advice, denying reality. The next psychiatrist also said the voice was that of my mother. I was forced to believe. What about you?

Since that time, I have worked with my mother and the psychiatrist to stop the inner voices. Essentially, this has worked. My relationship with mother is still fraught, with inappropriate power relations and other complications. However, the alternatives were to leave my family completely. I had tried moving to Adelaide but mother's voice came with me.

Finding my identity meant coming to know myself and my past. Learning emotional intelligence has been super empowering and allowed further self-awareness. It took practice, but it was SOOOO worth it, I am able to connect and engage, without panic, dissociation.

I cannot state strongly enough, always be aware of your inner connections. If you can be aware of your own inner emotional and intelligent life, then you can naturally engage with others in the 'universal' context. You will be aware, when someone asks you, internally, for help, or when you go for a job interview and the interviewer starts asking questions, 'in your head'. You can be in control, aware of your knowing authentic self.

Jenny Hickinbotham started writing before birth, via transference with her mother. Jenny experienced chronic child traumas and abuse, her grandmother told her she would write her story one day. Jenny has, written chapter and verse, here is another element. However, most with relevant power, like to keep people like Jenny, mental health challenges, silent. Jenny lives in Yarraville, Melbourne, with her two beautiful doggies, Puck and Trinky. Jenny's Blog is at: https://jennyhickinbotham.com/jens-blog. Thanks for connecting.

Gender and Redemption
Max Simensen

From as early as I can remember, I've been told that who I am, and
what I do, is wrong. Girls don't play with boy toys, wear boys' clothes,
do boy things. Gender stereotypes and roles were forced on me for as
long as I can remember. I used to scream and cry whenever I had to do
'girly' things, and the people around me thought that fighting gender
stereotypes was worse than my distress. I was very confused as a child as
to who I was and why I was built wrong. Society and the medical model
would say that I was born a girl, and that never fit with me. It scared and
challenged people in an unwanted way. A lot of people in my life would
rather I was unhappy than different.

I came out as a lesbian when I was 14 like it was the answer to an
algorithm: girl who likes girls = lesbian. I'd had people calling me a
lesbian, and other slurs, since I was 11, so I trusted others' judgment of
me more than my own. I was at a catholic school, which proved to be
a war zone for me. Bullying by other students and teachers throughout
my high school years tore away at my sense of self, and any self-esteem
societal standards left me with. From people yelling 'dyke' through
my classroom doorway to people physically hurting me in protest to
everything that I am and what I represented. When I'd reach out to
the teachers, I'd be told that my lifestyle was my choice and I had to
accept what came with it and if I did a little more repenting I might get
somewhere. I constantly had to fake a calm and confident demeanour so
people wouldn't see the emotional cracks forming in my exterior.

At the age of 14, when I came out as a lesbian, a cycle of abuse involving a family member started, and lasted for over five years: homophobia and disgust that came in the form of mental, emotional and physical abuse. I was told that I was nothing, broken, unnatural, and unlovable. These next five years shaped my mental health then and to this day. I was in survival mode, trying to get through the emotional turmoil that surrounded me. I felt nothing for years. I went from anger outbursts to dissociation, smashing walls to standing completely still looking off into the distance at nothing.

It took me years to understand that what happened to me was trauma and abuse. I feel that most people I've met who have been through trauma never feel like theirs is bad enough to talk about, particularly because so many people deep down feel that they deserved it, including me.

Through this time, I completely lost myself and developed a very deep, raw and active hatred of myself. I began to hate myself as much as everyone else hated me. Around this time, I met someone who was a trans man – a lightbulb went off in my head and I knew what I was. Everything connected and made sense. I'd heard how people spoke of trans people and the slurs used. I was terrified of who I was, and I knew that being a trans man would make an already hard situation unbearable. I didn't think I could live through that. At this point in my life, I would prefer ending my life over being a trans person. I had seen how trans people were treated and I couldn't handle it. I was half-way through my year 12 exams doing my trials when I decided this for myself. I went to school one day and wrote that I was trans in one of my English exams in the space for an essay as a final message to my teachers and students. Later that night I made an attempt at taking my own life and ended up alive in hospital on a mental health ward at the age of 17. I was ashamed, embarrassed and defeated.

At this point, I had a clinician from the local youth mental health team come and see me. This conversation changed the trajectory of the rest of my life. As a gay man, he spoke to me about trans people that he knew. He said, "If you're going to end your life anyway, why don't you try living one month as a boy and see how you go?" It seems simple, but I'd never thought of it that way. I may as well keep myself alive to trial it and see how I feel. From that point onwards, I made a commitment to myself to be Max. Max was going to be a powerful young man who fought through adversity. My mum made my transition and my mental health her full-time job, taking me to appointment after appointment to keep me alive. I began testosterone replacement therapy and my body started to change in a way that connected with me. Most people don't have to go through puberty a second time and the mood swings were torture. It wasn't easy by any stretch, but my mum had an unshakeable belief in my capacity and my future. We lived month to month for over a year.

During therapy I realised that a lot of the hurtful things that people did to me had pushed me to adapt my behaviour for survival. The anger, dissociation, self-harm and bottomless pit of reassurance I needed to be filled, were my main issues. My anger came from feeling unheard: the dissociation episodes were a sane reaction to insane circumstances in my life, the self-harm was a mix between an expression of pain and a cry for help, and realising that reassurance from other people was never going to be enough and I needed to give it to myself. Once I realised why I did those things, I was able to change them and curb episodes before I did toxic things to myself and others.

It's been tough, ugly, chaotic and torturous but the things that I've learned throughout these experiences have given me an innate skill to connect with other survivors and strugglers.

I began my first job as Max when I was 18 as a Mental Health Peer Worker at my local headspace. My role was to connect with other young people around distress and to be able to use genuine empathy to help soothe the wounds of others who had felt things like me. As soon as I began this role, I knew that I would do this for the rest of my life. My goal has been, and always will be, to be the person I needed when I was at my worst. I want to share and hold difficult emotional spaces with people who need it.

Fast forward, and I've been working as a Peer Worker, and on hormones for over five years. I have recently been employed in the position of Consumer Partnership Coordinator in South Eastern Sydney. I've moved away from my home town and am living in a house in Sydney with my partner and best friends. I stumbled across an extremely supportive group of friends who embrace who I am and constantly deal with my outbursts and chaos but love me through it every time.

I never thought I would make it to 23. I never thought my story would go past 18. There are so many people in my life who have held me through the really ugly times and I credit all that I am to them: to my friends who didn't know what to do or how to act, but still came to see me on the ward anyway and checked in on me often once I was out. I am actually content with my life and think about the future often. I've worked hard on accepting myself and letting myself be. Sometimes I have to agree to disagree with my self-hatred and try to inhabit my body with a treaty. Years of therapy have given me the foundation to grow into someone I can be proud of. I have built a career for myself that allows me to use my wounds to heal others. Turning my pain into something constructive and soothing for others has been most powerful for my recovery.

Some days are still really tough, and recovery isn't linear, but now I have an unshakeable belief in my capacity and my future.

I am Consumer Partnerships Coordinator for South Eastern Sydney Local Health District and work as an openly trans youth, LGBTIQA+ and mental health advocate. I've been a Peer Worker for over five years, a youth rep on the headspace National Youth Reference Group, a member of the Youth Advisory Council for Orygen (the National Centre of Excellence in Youth Mental Health) and a consumer representative on the Consumer Council for the Agency for Clinical Innovation.

Living with hope
Hope

My learning curve has led me to understand that recovery can only occur if we have real people in our lives buffered with a support system and meaningful activities. Chronic mental distress can lead to loss of family, friends, career, and normal social structure, whether that is environmentally, physically or emotionally. Many people come and go in our lives. Nobody can live our lives for us. Only we can find the right path that will help us feel a sense of belonging, or home within ourselves. We have to reconcile 'our lot in life' ourselves, by creating small victories and meaning in our lives. Moving closer to the notion of post-traumatic growth, I have had to settle for the feeling of something or someone, events, of being 'a good enough' fit. Ironically, even if this meant it was short-lived, not the perfect, sustaining place, or the people I wanted to evolve with as an end goal. I have learnt how to be resourceful, and kept seeking and researching ways to manage and bring about a sense of meaning and quality of life. This modified pathway helped me gain agency, a better understanding of myself and to feel connected to the rest of the world.

I have had to let go of searches for cures and accept that it is about living and managing one's experiences and intense feelings. I made the hard realisation that nobody has the answers. I have accepted that being sensitive is not a character flaw or pathology. It is a strength because it enables empathy and insight. One of the struggles I have worked through is knowing that I cannot control others' reactions or choices. If we are going to talk about extreme states and mental distress, then it forces me to include those same states from well meaning 'helpers'. I have been repeatedly abandoned, rejected, passed from one service to another, and re-traumatised by the very specialists claiming to know how to 'handle these presentations'. It is hard not to internalise those outcomes, asking if there is something faulty about one's self. I have lost count of all the half-skilled 'helpers' who have tried to 'crack the code'.

Even those 'experts' on others' lives, are trying to find their way home. In helping others, they feel out of their depth and flee from the greater risks that end up shining the torch on their own areas 'under construction'.

We are wired for fight and flight. We instinctively move towards things that make us feel safe and secure, and away from things that are contentious and uncertain.

Even 'specialist helping professionals' in 'inclusive' work places can lose boundaries and their moral compass. Anyone can be triggered if they feel criticised for their expert 'best efforts'. Unfortunately, those in the 'help industry' can cut off support, stigmatise and engage other tactics that misuse their positions of power. This makes life more challenging for those vulnerable to extreme states, resulting in exclusion, being cut-off from supports, powerlessness, loss of one's voice and having decision-making taken out of our hands.

It would be nice if others could keep in context one's suffering and trauma, and ask us what has happened rather than what is wrong. Instead of reacting, people in helping professions should exercise compassion and work from a framework that values humanity. There can be strong and rigid reactions to personalities that people fear or do not want to take time to understand. It has been an overused tactic to use the 'mentally ill' as the political guinea pig. It becomes formulaic when reputations or jobs have been on the line by using stereotypical labels such as 'safety risk', the 'unhinged client' or 'the typical angry borderline'. Stereotypes are perpetuated when 'help' professionals profile their clients based on 'the text-book typical type of conduct'. Stereotyping is self-serving, at the price of other people's gain. We 'disorders' lose credibility, it's hard to be heard and believed against the more 'normal' presentation of the 'well-integrated' person.

Understanding my experience of distress and finding a pathway through

Instrumental in making sense of myself and the world was understanding that many of us have had some variation and themes on a spectrum of lived experience, instead of seeing myself singled out like some broken machinery. The common thread of the human condition is that most of us have had adversity in our lives. This has made me feel less isolated. While we are alive on the planet we feel, and this has an impact, a consequence – behavioural and social effects.

In my search for restoration and repair, in seeking a sense of 'home', tribe, and trying to be a contributing part of society, there has not been a lot of 'ways forward' on offer. Suffering seems to be a big pathologised industry and there seems to be a pool of experts and PhD's and intellectual prowess in human science. However, I have not come across many in the field who encourage disclosure of concentrated ongoing levels of trauma and lived experience of multiple extreme adversities.

Contributing factors to my lived experience include cultural dislocation – leaving one's genetic home and familiar surroundings. The removal from and loss of tribe and language were often overlooked by helping professionals. In hindsight, I learnt these factors triggered extreme states and the ability to form my own cultural identity. Another is the disruption of developmental stages – because of poverty, living in orphanages, prolonged neglect, constant lack of supervision and abandonment, intergenerational child abuse and violence, bullying. These are extreme states for the brain and the body to process.

It is possible to find one's way over time. Sadly, what I have observed though is that often it seems unfamiliar for those in or out of the profession to know how to accept those with 'complex presentations' from infancy to adulthood. Most events occur across a life span, not all at once, for lengthy protracted passages of time. The more that happens the longer your brain needs to redevelop, rewire and regulate.

Longer term embedded trauma is more challenging to integrate back to the routine and structure of the expected 'normal' socially acceptable life. The 'experts' seem unsure of what to make of the presentation of duality: one of intense super sensitivity, overreactions and dysregulation; and one of demonstrating rational, articulate, insightful, 'high functioning' attributes to the extent of being just as skilled and astute as 'the experts'.

Turning point

A significant turning point for me was when I got more interested in learning about human science and humanistic education. Around this time, I was introduced to peer work and the value and strength of lived experience. I have seen how these attributes have exacted change and contributed to breaking down old myths and barriers in one's thoughts and actions.

Meaningful connections and actions

Placing importance on being proactive and engaging in personal development education has led me to meet like-minded people. Education has generated some profound and validating conversations in hearing others' stories, creating some distance and perspective. An unexpected consequence has been that I was then able to support and impart my learning and my resources with others who were in the dark about directions and had similar struggles in their recovery.

Psycho-education has been validating but cognition alone will not help heal neural pathways. Movement of the body, of any kind, also aids self-regulation. People with a nervous disposition may display nervous movements such as an inability to sit still. Stereotypes are perpetuated because people may cast doubt on one's 'wellness'. These movements should be affirmed as positive, the wisdom of the body expelling the trauma and signs of the body resourcing itself.

While I have done much self-rebuilding on my own, and felt years of isolation, I have had pockets of meaningful connection through friends and chance meetings. These rare few stuck by and looked beyond the labels. It's helped hearing shared stories and similar journeys at events and collaborative projects. These relationships have assisted me to remain integrated in the world.

Volunteer gardening has made me feel a part of a productive group. This community garden also has an education centre which has given me the opportunity to attend free courses on sustainable leadership, organic gardening, bee keeping and animal/husbandry studies. I have found enjoyment in permaculture expos, film nights and guest speaker talks.

Music is also rewarding and a source of healing. For instance, exploring the community to play piano in hospitals. This year, I made a commitment to have more fun, so I have been out going to plays, comedy events and laughing more often. I have felt moments of happiness sitting in the city following the busker's shift and soaking up their musical talents, forgetting myself for a moment or two. I guess I live in hope.

'Hope' is nearly hitting mid 40's and has lived experience of CPTSD. Hope has lived overseas in Canada & Africa, originally adopted from overseas but raised in white bread Australia by a white privileged cultural family. Loves playing the piano, into yoga, meditation, reading, walks in nature and by the beach. Enjoys learning and attending trauma informed care and personal development workshops. Currently Hope is doing a Certificate II in Community Service and Peer Work.

To my Eating Disorder
Jessica Leask

To my Eating Disorder,

I want to completely get rid of you for good, I don't want my life dictated by you and your rules anymore.

You have lied to me, taken away so much, warped my sense of reality in more ways than one, isolated me and tormented me for over 10 years. You become stronger on and off, win many battles and send me packing for hospital. However, I am determined that you will not win this war and that my latest hospital admission was the last.

You are there every day – at my meal times two to three times a day, when I catch a glimpse of myself in a mirror or reflective surface, when I'm getting dressed, taking a shower, reading the menu at restaurants or cafés, at my therapy appointments when I'm talking about how to overcome you, when exercising at the gym and when lying in bed at night going over what I have eaten that day and then making promises to you that I will eat less, lose weight and get to a size you are happy with. At the moment, the thought of having to deal with you at least six times a day while 'implementing an adequate meal plan' is extremely terrifying.

Right now, food is the enemy. I don't crave it, enjoy it, prepare it, look forward to it. I'm never hungry, even since I increased my exercise. I truly believe my life would be a lot easier if food weren't part of it. But that hasn't always been the way. I remember a time when I would cook.

My speciality was lemon meringue pie and the best part was eating it.
I haven't cooked that in many years despite requests from my family to
do so. I would eat McDonalds straight after exerting myself at dance
class on a Friday night, my standard order a Big Mac meal with a large
chocolate sundae. I would look forward to that meal all week and the
thought of how many calories were in it, or how I would later compensate
for having eaten it did not even enter my mind. You were not part of my
life, I was carefree, confident, a fun person to be around (I hope) and
most importantly, happy. I hope I come to fully realise that food is not the
enemy and that you are!

You have taken away so much from me. My university experience,
supposed to be the time of my life, was spent battling you at your
strongest. Logging all my food on the computer, exercising compulsively,
then entering the exercise and seeing the number of calories I'd consumed
drop, was my highlight. It gave me a rush, a sense of achievement, a
distraction from everything else. You later put me in hospital multiple
times, taking me away from the thing I care about most – my dog, Metta.
You made me compare myself to other girls, made me think that I didn't
deserve or need to be there because I was bigger than most of them.

You have made and continue to make me think that because I am not
thin, not the typical age of a sufferer (you started in adulthood rather
than adolescence), and that I don't have the more talked about diagnoses,
that you are not serious enough or that I am not sick enough to warrant
treatment. That I don't have the diagnosis of anorexia and am not at
a low weight, you tell me I have failed – that I even suck at having an
eating disorder. Your voice says I'm 'not bad enough, so keep trying and
get worse'. You tell me that obviously I'm not a strong person because
I am actually consuming food, and that many of your more successful

followers don't even do that, and that's what makes you happiest and most proud!

But you are all consuming. I've lost friendships. I've been told by friends that it's too hard to hold a conversation with me when I'm not eating properly. I guess my head gets too caught up in you. Many of my friends haven't been able to understand how you work and they think that all I need to do to overcome you is to *just* eat. If only it were that simple!

In the past, you have taken away jobs and my psychology internship. Now I've fallen into being a Peer Support Worker and absolutely love my work. But people are telling me you will take that away from me too if I continue to listen to and obey you. However, though I hear it from other people, you keep whispering in my ear to make me believe that things will never get that bad, that I can have an eating disorder and be a Peer Worker at the same time. If I think about it, I can try to challenge your voice by remembering my past attempts to hold down a job whilst maintaining an eating disorder – I have the evidence that the two cannot co-exist or at least haven't yet in my case. But still your voice keeps telling me it'll never get that bad – I'm still functioning fine, this time it's different.

But functioning could be more than just getting to places on time. It could be getting through an entire day without crying. It could be going out to a restaurant or café without panicking and being distracted by the foods on the menu and instead just enjoying the company and conversations. Or functioning could be spontaneously having an ice cream on a hot day to cool down. It could be not watching the clock all day everyday dreading the countdown to the next time I have to eat. It could be not counting the calories of everything I put into my mouth, or working my muscles to capacity during gym class to make sure I am burning off as many calories as possible. I think functioning effectively in life is being able to get full pleasure out of what life has to offer, being present, and being able to get enjoyment out of, or at least just regularly and adequately consume, the one thing that keeps you alive – which is food.

You lie to me but make it sound like the truth. You twist my mind and thoughts, especially when my treatment team tell me something that goes against what you believe. You twist their words to make it sound like their words apply to everyone else except me, or that they are the ones lying to me. Then you make me lie to people, with the excuse they are 'just little white lies which won't hurt anybody'. But these little white lies do hurt somebody – me. Now I'm done with lying, I am going to tell the truth because no one can help me get over you for good if I don't be strong, ignore what you want me to say, and instead say what's really going on with me physically and mentally.

You point out every flaw I have, you tell me I'm not good enough and make me think I am worthless. In the past you have stopped at nothing – taking away my jobs, internship, friends. You stopped me from enjoying my 20s and you put me in hospital many times when all I wanted was to lose a few kilos. You are beginning to do those things again, yet I continue to listen to you.

I don't want my life to be all about food, the number of calories in a banana, the amount of calories I can burn off during exercise or the size of the clothes I can fit into. I want to be able to cook for myself. I want to be a successful peer worker. I want to be an amazing aunty and be a role model to my niece, Eliza and my nephew, Hugh. I want to go back overseas once I can save up enough money. I want to be healthy and happy for Metta. I want to be a laid-back sister and daughter, so my family can relax and don't feel they have to tip-toe around me anymore. I want to go out to restaurants and cafes for delicious meals with friends. I want to make those trying to help me proud of me and most importantly I want to make the most of my 30's and create new memories in which you aren't featured at all. I want to leave you. I want my life to be filled with laughter and not tears, with friends and not loneliness and with health and not fear.

You will probably always follow me like a shadow continually whispering in my ear. I'm sure you will always try to trick me and catch me off guard when I am vulnerable. But I want to have the strength and ability to confront you, then turn my back on you and eventually have your voice just as a passing thought. I have heard from others that this is possible, and I desperately want that to be the case for me.

So yes, eating disorder, although you are winning many of the battles with me at the moment, and have become stronger and more present, I can still remember the time you weren't in my life. This gives me hope that can again be the case. So, I will listen to the people who really care about me and have my best interests at heart and I will believe them over you, so I can one day stand proud and tell people that yes, I did have an eating disorder, but that fight is over. I want to be able to say the most significant battle in my life has been won through sheer guts, determination and the ability to accept and believe that I deserve and am worthy of the help and support I am currently receiving.

Jessica graduated from UOW with a Postgraduate Diploma in Psychology but due to becoming unwell was unable to complete her registration. Years later she completed the Cert-IV Mental Health Peer Work qualification, has since worked as a Peer Support Worker and values sharing her living experience of mental health concerns with the clients she meets. Jessica is also a huge dog lover and keeps well by spending time with her own Maltese X Shih Tzu baby.

My Partner Forgot About Our Relationship, Here's What Happened Next
Grace Hoffman

Or so a clickbait article would be titled if I was a lazy writer. This forgetting of a relationship was part 50 First Dates, part Eternal Sunshine of the Spotless Mind, part Memento but not nearly as cool but still a little bit thrilling.

So the person who I was in a relationship with forgot that we had been in a relationship. This was a direct result of electroconvulsive therapy, ECT, shock therapy. Memory loss is one of the more notable effects. ECT these days, is less One Flew Over the Cuckoo's Nest and more something out a Foucauldian nightmare. A nightmare with more routine, which is more normalised, more operational, but with the much of the same debilitating side effects.

How did we get to a point where a person is getting ECT and a relationship has been forgotten?

I remember it every time I go to the supermarket. This is because I was in that supermarket when I received a heart-breaking message that marked the start of that journey. I am buying the exact same things I used to every week, two tins lentils, two tins tomatoes, two tins chickpeas, two kilos fruit, one almond milk, one soy. I'm stealing much of these from the self-serve checkout when I get a text message which I check after I exit the store. It is a message that I know right away means the person I care for has tried to end their life.

Two days later, I am raising my voice and gesticulating at a nurse after I am told off for showing too much physical affection. I'm telling them that I should be allowed to hug the person I care for when they are in a psychiatric hospital.

Two days later they are discharged to go home and have agreed to undertake ECT.

That I feel responsible for them undertaking ECT is influenced by my narcissism, but I know that I actually *am* responsible in some small way. This is because I had said to them that I have heard of and known many people who experience what gets called treatment resistant depression who have had ECT, and have found the experience to be very beneficial, and who had limited side effects.

They begin ECT.

In the coming weeks, I visit them many days each week and it becomes apparent to me that something is a bit different. In an attempt to create shared optimism for the future, I mention a possible future where we live together. They tell me that they don't think we have that kind of relationship. I think I'm being told that we are not, and cannot, be lovers anymore. What I am actually being told is that they don't remember that we have been in an intimate relationship.

In this period, I can see the gaps in their memory, I can see that new memories are not being stored. They come over and ask me when I got a new fridge again and again and again. Every time I see them I make sure to tell them the same joke:

What's the best thing about telling jokes to someone getting ECT? You can tell them the same one over and over and over again.

I told this a couple of times until the seriousness of the situation made it all very unfunny.

I go to visit them and mostly in silence we watch the 24-hour ABC news channel all day. I want to sit close to them, wrap my arms around them, kiss them, but I have got the message and continue to get the message, that it is not appropriate given my perception of our new dynamic. Of course though, people I care about deserve love and support independent of the nature of the relationship, so I keep visiting. What has been happening changes nothing, I still love them deeply.

We are completing a puzzle that is inspired by The Starry Night by Vincent van Gogh. You'd know the painting, the one with the stars and swirls. There is nothing I would rather be doing less than this fucking puzzle. I leave that day and catch the train home sobbing, listening to the song 'Vincent' by Don McLean. You would know that one too, it's about a starry starry night.

Two days later I am holding onto the leash of an enormous greyhound. They are visiting their local area mental health service whilst I am holding onto this dog which they had recently adopted. They have also at one point, post a treatment, forgotten they have a dog.

I am very scared that this greyhound will somehow get off the leash and run away and everything will be ruined. However, the dog does not run away. Then, they drive us home. I don't drive, I am scared of driving.

As we are driving they mention how I should 'totally date' one of their close friends. I remain quiet and churning with frustration because I had intended and was until recently 'totally dating' *them*. Ever the empath, they can tell some part of me is upset so they enquire. I say, "I don't want to date them, I want to be dating *you*".

My attempts of recreating intimacy and a closeness again miss the mark, they don't really understand and now they feel like I am inappropriately trying to put the moves on them during an incredibly difficult time in their life. Maybe I was.

ECT continues. ECT is over. Some joy has been unearthed in their previously blank looking face. They bang on my mouldy apartment door, they come in with enthusiasm. Something is different. I'm thrilled.

Weeks go by and we are friendly and talk often. I am selfish, I'm heart broken. I love you. I've told you this and you've told me the same thing, but it's somehow missing.

I remember the times that we first spent with each other, our first date, kiss, fuck. They don't.

I'm not sure what to do with those memories. Memory can be considered a source of knowledge, providing that someone is there to bear witness to it as evidence or justification of them. These memories sometimes feel a little incomplete now. I am saddened that these memories only exist in my head but I am so glad they are there to share with them.

Time passes. They have uncovered some but not all of the memories. Through much effort we begin to remember each other together. We paint ourselves into each other's lives again. I still love them. They love me too. We live together now. We make new memories, rediscover the old ones and do our best to lessen the shackles of madness. It's humorous and awful. It's a plot befitting a film or novel, just not one I would ever watch or read.

Recently I have held the title for the crazier of the two of us. This is because I have spent some time in hospital. Recently my case manager asked me "have you considered ECT?" The answer is yes, but only so we can be even.

Grace dreams of a better world.
"We carry a new world here, in our hearts. That world is growing this minute." – Durruti

Untitled
Richard Affleck

Daddy was an engineer and Mommy was a housewife of military bearing, living the 1950s American Dream. Uncompromisingly conventional, they believed in routine and discipline, precision and regularity. (They purchased Dr Spock, not to read it, but because it was a best-seller.) Childrearing was easy: predictability was the key. So, when in 1953 I had a difficult and ill-timed birth, my mother, proud of her childbearing prowess, held me responsible. It was a bad start, and kept getting worse.

The dark side of their big dream was their emotional and physical volatility. After all, they were both survivors of severe childhood trauma.

It was hard on them, I imagine, me forcing them to beat me because of my chaotic, dreamy, wandering nature, which disrupted their schedules and confounded their theories.

Nevertheless, I seemed a happy little kid. In the classroom photos from kindergarten I was always beaming, always full of life. I have no memories of the school, but my report card said I was a pleasure to teach because I had a *good mind.*

I was an optimist in those days. I ran away, not because of the beatings, but because I was off to California where the sun always shines. Well, that Kalamazoo wasn't waiting for me in the Chicago railyards, so I had to return and face the music.

When we emigrated to Australia things got worse. Mum was lonely and homesick and took it out on us. My new school was a strange, dangerous place, full of 'orphans' – stolen and rejected children – and steeped in violence. The male teachers were sadistic thugs. It didn't help that I was short-sighted and autistic.

I'll spare you the details, but insist on the constancy of stress, and of fear, and of anger and grief and confusion. They were what I would have to recover from: a wreck of a life that rendered me a wreck of a man.

Scilicet: I was a damned fool throughout.

The culmination and terminus of my grand cavalcade of shit occurred in 2003, in a government job where I was subjected to sexual harassment, coordinated persecution, scapegoating and criminal defamation. Uncharacteristically, I tried to defend myself, but I failed, and when I failed I fell apart, and so did my life. This, I propose, was the beginning of my recovery, which began in or around 2003 and continues to this day. Let me enumerate its elements. Dates are approximate.

June 2003: I went to a psychologist for stress counselling, but was promptly shuffled down the hall to the psychiatrist's office, where one Dr Fishbein decided I was bipolar and wanted to put me on lithium; so I ran away. (I'm on lithium now and rather like it.) But here was an answer to an old question: those rare days, scattered through my life, when for no reason everything seemed quite alright. Well, it turns out those days were pathological, hypomania, to be precise, little bubbles of happiness rising up through my swamp of melancholy.

Soon after that, I went for another opinion to Dr Flanagan. He sat me down to a series of personality inventories. Look, he said, you score 39 out of 50 on the Dissociative Experiences Scale. Thirty-one is the cutoff for Dissociative Identity Disorder (DID) You have DID. Oh. Pennies dropped like raindrops. Who was I?

September 2003: Around the time of my breakdown (for I suppose that is what it was) I moved from the suburbs to a flat in Katoomba, where half the population seemed to be mad. I proceeded to get involved in community theatre, playback theatre, theatre sports. I made new friends, wrote and recorded music. At the same time, however, I was not doing well. I and my life were out of control. Money disappeared. I drank heavily and ran through my flat night after night, tearing at my clothes, smashing things, shouting at my captors. Maybe the drugs weren't working.

Then I found psychotherapist Linda. She faithfully conducted me back through the workplace episode, back through all those terrible workplaces, and back through my childhood, picking up the pieces. She said she sometimes saw 40 alters in play.

Our work lasted years and must have integrated me to a degree. The parts may have come together but fracture lines remain, lines of weakness under stress. What kind of man do they add up to, anyway? My vision was that of a teacher, tired and apprehensive, as she surveys a schoolyard…

Linda told me: survivors of childhood abuse are marked out forever. They send subliminal signals which can easily be detected by dangerous adults. Thus, the mysterious phenomenon of *adult revictimisation:* I had a sign on my back saying: *kick me.*

2004-5: I wrote a book of 1800 pages. It was about everything and nothing and had no title. Linda encouraged me.

[I]deology represents itself in all its versions as an uncomplicated, unambiguous entity – an unfolded plane, an unknotted thread, a solid object standing only for itself. 'You see, it's all quite simple', it smiles. The rest is furious casuistry, art concealing art.

And so on. My father told me I was a fool to waste my time on this rubbish, as if I were bloody Karl Marx. Anyway, it now lies *dishabille*, accumulating the dust of irrelevance, a monument to my boundless enthusiasm. But you see, I was actually *writing,* writing for the first time in a sustained and semi-systematic way.

In 2004 I got onto the Disability Support Pension (DSP), thanks to Dr. Flanagan's letter. Without the pension… well, the pension made possible my recovery, such as it is. Without it I would have become homeless.

In or around 2009 a mad friend in Katoomba recommended his own psychiatrist, Dr Fred Smith, a true wizard with the drugs; and sure enough, after some preliminary fumbles, Fred did get me sorted out. I now take seven medications. (But then, is this the real me?)

I have always seen and heard music in my head, and have been idly writing it down for over 50 years, like doodling. I mentioned this to Dr Smith. He asked me if I could write a symphony... well, it took me five years, on and off, writing about myself, in music, as honestly as I could. Hardly anyone thought it was any good, but at least this time nobody called me a liar or a cheat.

In 2011, I got a part-time job as a support worker with Aftercare. I made friends, had a great boss, did a pretty OK job of it. I loved it there. The problems of others gave me time away from my own. But one night, after three years of this, the angel of death landed on my shoulder and instructed me to leave and finish the symphony. And so I did, in 2015.

My recovery manifested itself in my life in the world – not just a private affair of sanity and madness, but something that amounted to an emergence into the light, in the company of others.

Let me tell you about some of these others. For four years plus, I have been seeing Sharon Jones (not the singer), a clever, nimble and vaguely angelic being, my sixth psychiatrist. This work has changed me fundamentally, in a good way. Sharon says I have *matured* over that time. I am more concerned with love now, more aware of its place in my life. But that is another story.

In 2017, I rejoined Blue Mountains Playback Theatre in Katoomba. There we improvise re-enactments of stories told by audience members. I've gotten pretty good at slipping into somebody's skin, no matter whose. When the magic is up, my body disappears, to be replaced by that of someone much younger, and my mind… my mind steps back, tired and apprehensive, and watches. There is an uncluttered void at my centre, you know, nothingness, freedom. Anything might happen… but things work out in the moment. That, I think, is what it is to be alive.

None of this would be possible without the trust that holds us all together in Playback, trust that has liberated me from my old paralysing performance anxiety. With their help, I have crossed an ancient threshold of fear. The anthropologist Victor Turner wrote that threshold and fear are integral parts of the ritual process. Without these there is no transformation. And without the group there is no ritual, no suspension of disbelief, and no show.

It has proven useful to be married to a trauma specialist. Sandra Warn has pulled me together more than once. She has the dirt on me.

Have I recovered? If I had, how would I know it? Should I be happy? Should I be calm? Should I be setting myself some concrete goals? Ha! But surely, recovery is not a destination, but an open winding path, an alternative to the tight little circles into which we might be persuaded to train our lives…

I'm working on an opera now.

Born: 1953, Cleveland Ohio, USA.
1961: Immigrated to Australia.
Attended schools in Chicago, Denver, Sydney and Melbourne.
Degrees from Sydney University (Arts) and UNE (Psychology)
Drama training: Ensemble Theatre, Q Theatre, Drama Action Centre.
Jobs: numerous, mostly menial – factory hand, cleaner, public servant, welfare worker, support worker, TAFE teacher, etc. I 'retired' in 2015.

I write words. I write music. Big deal.

An EXTREMITY leading to new life orientation.
Spiritual Awakening...and deepening crisis enmeshed in the Bipolar state
Catherine Conroy

A new 'force' awoke within me in 2000. With something of the same Icarus speed I'd known the 'heightened state' of ecstatic revelry and 'spiritual' joy to arise... came the THUD... Fear wrapped a shroud of deadly anguish around me.

Terrifyingly and utterly.

For years, the events surrounding my deepest experience of darkness remained mysterious. The sense of horrifying dread in reality and upon reflection filled my mind and heart and I had great difficulty understanding the meaning of the 'spiritually' dark experience of personal chaos.

On a beautiful day in 2000 having recently completed six years of mental health consumer advocacy, I visited friends. We talked and prayed together. At that time, full of fervour, my reference was St. Paul and with determination I put on the whole armour of God.

> *"So stand ready, with truth as a belt tight around your waist, with righteousness as your breastplate, and as your shoes the readiness to announce the Good News of peace.*
> *At all times carry faith as a shield, for with it you will be able to put out all the burning arrows shot by the evil one.*
> *And accept salvation as a helmet and the word of God as a sword **which the spirit gives you.**"[1]*

---

1 *St. Paul's Letter to the Ephesians 6:13-17*

At the time, I had fight in my being and an emotional stance professing myself strongly against the 'devil'.

In the sun, I left my friends' house to walk home experiencing a strange 'crack' in my head.

With fear that day too, I identified some frightening phenomena. I had a mental battle whilst showering, trembling greatly and trying to ward off an incessant feeling, pushing against me. I had to fight. Later in the day, calmer and whilst listening to music, a visionary event depicting myself in a boat sailing into a cave, occurred. The following day I was at home by myself and while reading an old assignment related to the 'Future' something very strange happened. The news broadcast stopped suddenly on the name Slobodan Milošević.

The next clear events were shocking. I recall a sense of what I believe to be an experience of the Precious Blood. I was literally led from our house into the park which is just opposite our home. Close to the rose garden I instantaneously crouched down and at once I was psychically beaten and internally pulverised... I was in the deepest fear, unbelievably lashed, scathed and bashed. I felt unrelentingly spiritually and emotionally apprehended.

I returned to our house in a deeply shocked blur, stunned, and in total disarray. I felt myself assailed by a moving shroud of darkness. In terror, I tried to phone my parents but the phone wouldn't work.

I raced upstairs, my legs shaking violently. I was engulfed in unimaginable fear and loathing. Suffering was the understanding... the word for my whole being.

My mother had given me a heavy gold cross and I grasped it now. My acute desperation gradually dissipated.

For the rest of that year I was unable to work. In fact, I could do very little. I cried nearly every day, filled with doom and sorrow. I was very lonely, very lost...my whole person in pieces, a sense of great loss, my moorings shot from under me. I was in a place of dark and deep unknown. A melancholy and grief unlike all other experiences besieged me. At the time, I felt ripped asunder from God.

Many years passed as I tried to understand. A lot of the time I felt God was punishing me. Often, I felt deeply angry with God. Frightened of Him too. How could He allow something like this to happen? I was positively bereft. Why did something like this ever take place? It was all so hard for me to understand, especially considering the glorious and gorgeous experiences I had had of God.

> *"Death could scarce be more bitter than that place!*
> *But since it came to good, I will recount*
> *all that I found revealed there by God's grace."*[2]

I began to think perhaps, in an inexplicable way, that a head injury and unresolved post-traumatic stress, a subsequent bipolar diagnosis triggered by prescribed diet medication, and a post-partum psychosis contributed in part, to the experience. As well, there'd been some substantial 'growing up' dilemmas. I recall very vividly one day towards the end of my advocacy work, the sense and sound of inpatient doors banging and closing deeply 'within'. Strange.

---

2 *Dante A. (1555) The Inferno, The Divine Comedy, Gabrielle Giolito de' Ferrari.*

At this time, I was unknowing, not acknowledging anything of the critical 'inner voice' and 'inner passivity'... the language of the defensive process, sometimes hostile towards others and said to be the core of 'maladaptive' behaviour.

To be medicated and to remain medicated for decades has been precarious and devastating, truly 'through a glass darkly'[3]. To feel at the time a 'perception' of the grace of God removed, was beyond recognition.

My journey became a deep quest for understanding. I searched high and low. Sometimes obsessively.

With the deeply thoughtful and most helpful navigation of a spiritual counsellor I undertook a 'Life Healing Journey'[4] retreat, which offered an understanding of the stages of grieving as a kind of 'cognitive life-raft' – an assurance that feelings are normal.

Most importantly for me, the workbook at the time, contained a scriptural model of spirituality that looked at 'The Spirituality of the Heart' – healing distorted images of God, false images of God, and living the mystery of suffering.

I was guided too, at this time and over the years, to understand the ways in which writing helps to surface what we hold locked up in our unconscious... the denials, anger, bargaining, sadness, unforgiveness, attachments, the way shame and guilt can get into the way of healing and covenant... the life-long healing journey...

A Jungian therapist sustained sound direction for me and I began to

---

3 *Biblical phrase, 1 Corinthians 13:12*
4 *Fr. Peter E. Campbell MSC (2010) co-founder of "Life's Healing Journey: A Path to Peace."*

explore dream symbols which are sparse. For some time after receiving the Blessed Sacrament, a flower would 'appear.' That always gave me great joy and I was reminded of the words of Saint Exupery in 'The Little Prince': "One sees clearly only with the heart. Anything essential is invisible to the eyes"[5]. A beautiful relationship was being created.

"Thanks to the human heart by which we live,
Thanks to its tenderness, its joys, and fears..."[6]

While doing some serious inner child healing work, remnants of my childhood emerged. Great emotional soothing and revelation. 'I have a little shadow' the R. L. Stephenson poem, once memorised, suddenly received my attention with brand new eyes! Until the garden 'awakening', my unknown shadow side indeed was the dramatic and unexpected and unprecedented, most painful opening I believe, of my unconscious... and perhaps collective unconscious. That began my commitment to my spiritual journey and to doing the extraordinarily profound work that began within me. I believe in originally being "knitted together in my mother's womb."[7] ... "And the vision that was planted in my brain ... still remains ..."[8]

"Our birth is but a sleep and a forgetting:
The Soul that rises with us, our life's Star,
Hath had elsewhere its setting,
And cometh from afar:
Not in entire forgetfulness,
And not in utter nakedness,
But trailing clouds of glory do we come
From God, who is our home ..."[9]

---

5 Antoine de Saint Exupery (1955) "The Little Prince" Wordsworth Editions Limited 1995.

6 William Wordsworth (1807) "Intimations of Immortality from Recollections of Early Childhood."

7 Psalm 139: 13-14 New International Version (NIV) 4th Edition (2011).

8 Paul Simon (1964) "The Sounds of Silence."

9 William Wordsworth (1807) "Intimations of Immortality from Recollections of Early Childhood."

Praying for a journey of healing and receiving some vision, I began to comprehend what has been and remains fundamentally challenging and even evolutionary... the true movement towards CONSCIOUSNESS and self-acceptance along the way. My most important and ongoing spiritual gift of hope and understanding, enables me to experience unconditional love, divine love. "When unconditional love comes forward as our new organizing principle, our innate spiritual power and dignity arises, and we can no longer be so shaken by life's circumstances."

Miraculously, and in a tangible way, the hypomanic and depressive states have considerably evened out, apart from a hospitalisation in 2013 with lithium toxicity, and the passing of my mother.

Following some devastating falls at that time and loss of mobility, I recently had a hip replacement. Although my equilibrium was quite sorely challenged, I believe the extraordinary experience of conversion... "unconscious becoming conscious", the steady opening up to my soul, and the ongoing clear work of the journey to individuation provides for me, a true sense that fulfilment and happiness can reside.

Along with the support of my loving family, my spiritual director, and spiritual healing, 'The Life Healing Journey' has been of inestimable worth to me, a marvellous turning point in my life... providentially there.

Notwithstanding, the many rocky roads I have been able to identify and navigate with help, a truly worthwhile and meaningful inner journey, trusting that God well knows the huge mortal storms.

> *"And I said to the man who stood at the gate of the year:*
> *'Give me a light that I may tread safely into the unknown.'*

And he replied:
'Go out into the darkness and put your hand into the Hand of God.
That shall be to you better than light and safer than a known way.'
So I went forth, and finding the Hand of God, trod gladly into the night.
And He led me towards the hills and the breaking of day in the lone
East." [10]

So, heart be still.

A baby boomer, born 1952, just as Britain tested the first atomic bomb.
Later the Beatles were singing "Love me Do," Martin Luther King saying,
"I have a dream." Setting out from Dry Plains, Adaminaby to seek my
fortune...my lifelong love and I had 3 children...and now there are 4
grandchildren. As teachers there has been wonderful life opportunities
alongside a dose of adversity.

---

10 *Minnie Louise Haskins (1908) "The Gate of the Year", "God Knows".*

What's Your Superpower?
Livonne Larkins

What's your superpower? I discovered mine when I was about three. A superpower that has saved me from many perils. A superpower that has rescued me from trauma. A superpower that has kept me more balanced than I really have any right to be. My superpower is being able to step outside of myself. Let me tell you more about how this came about.

I'm the 11th of 12 children, so life was always chaotic. My parents took me to a doctor when I was about three years old as I was 'highly strung' and always crying. In fact my family nickname was 'Cry-baby' or the 'Waterworks', and I refused to eat anything much other than cornflakes so I was considered a spoilt brat by my siblings. The doctor put me on a tonic, but what the doctor and my parents didn't realise is that I was being sexually abused by a family member.

Around the same time, amidst the trauma, something magical happened. Someone gave us a 'read along' book of Mary Poppins. It had a vinyl record with it that you played as you read, and Tinkerbell rang a bell, when it was time to turn the page. This bit of bliss was how I learned to read and so escape abuse, in my own childlike way.

So I learned to read well before I started school and I began to separate myself from the little girl who was being abused. Oh, I felt sorry for her but while she was suffering I was climbing The Magic Faraway Tree with Dame Washalot and Moonface. Or I was having a tea-party on the ceiling with Mary Poppins, Uncle Bert and Michael and Jane Banks. I was swimming with mermaids and flying high with fairies.

As I got a bit older, I became part of the Secret Seven and Famous Five, or I was wandering through the property of Misrule with the children from Seven Little Australians. The abuse continued but my superpower kicked in, and I escaped into imagination. It helped me to function in everyday life.

I grew up more normal than I probably deserved to be, got married and had my first baby, a little girl called Aimee. She was followed closely by Lachlan and Stuart. The four of us revelled in fantasy. I taught them all my favourite songs like Puff the Magic Dragon, and Emerald City. We watched everything Disney and everything not Disney, as long as it piqued our imaginations. We were thrilled to lose ourselves in the toy box in Andy's room in Toy Story, or swim under the sea with Ariel in The Little Mermaid. We were a family inspired by fantasy.

I became unhappy in my marriage, however I started acting in amateur theatre and lost myself in the thrill of it. Watching a scene come to life fascinated me: the words, costumes, props, sets. It was another form of magic. The marriage became violent and ultimately ended. Then my ex-husband stalked, harassed and terrorised us. For over four years, I was living on about two hours of sleep a night; working full time, mothering traumatised children, and spending massive amounts of time in court, as the harassment and violence got worse.

Without realising it, I started to step outside the situation – as I had as a child. I was better able to cope with being responsible for the kids when I removed all emotion from the situation. I saw it all as if I was a third party to the assaults. When I was woken in the middle of the night, with kids being dragged out of windows, I was usually able to react without emotion. My superpower to the rescue.

After many years of this – one night – the unthinkable happened. Three children went on an access visit but only two came home.

My beautiful Aimee gained her angel wings that night. My boys were both badly injured but would live, thank God. Not knowing how to cope with the pain of grief, I once again stepped outside the situation. I threw myself back into acting and for a few hours each week it was bliss, as I became someone else, and the pain didn't exist. The moment I stepped off stage, the pain was back and emotionally I was crippled.

Only three years later, I held my beautiful mum in my arms as she crossed to a kinder shore. Again, I had to step away from the emotion of losing the two most important girls in my life, my mother and my daughter, but it was getting harder to find ways to step outside of myself. This time, my superpower was nowhere to be found.

That's when I discovered a chat room on the internet. I was able to hide behind a screen and be someone else for a few hours each night. No one knew how broken I was. I was able to play a role again but this time no one could see the pain in my eyes. I developed a new persona named Livonne. She was so much more confident and funny than me. She was my superpower at its best, but I controlled her. As the years went by, we grew more like each other. She became a bit more serious and I became a bit more outgoing. The lines between us blurred.

Over time, the boys grew older as boys do, the chat room had closed down and I no longer acted.

One day I was driving with Lachlan in the car, when I forgot what to do. By this stage I had been driving for about 22 years so driving had become part of muscle memory, but I completely forgot what I was supposed to be doing. Lachlan who had his learners permit, realised something was wrong, and helped me pull the car over. He put his L plates on and drove me home. That's when I was diagnosed with Complex PTSD.

I was seriously depressed, anxiety held me captive: the slightest noise could trigger my PTSD and the only thing holding me to this life was my sons. As much as I wanted to go and be with Aimee, I didn't want to leave my boys. My life was completely in ruins. I couldn't hold a job down and was embarrassed at having been diagnosed with a mental illness, as I saw it as a sign of weakness. My mind was too overwhelmed to find a way of stepping out of itself. So I ran away.

I made a new life for myself in the Blue Mountains in NSW, going back to study to keep myself busy. If there was a course on offer that was free, I did it. One of these was an introduction to Fine Art. I had always been crafty but art wasn't my best subject at school so didn't think it would be for me. Surprisingly, I really loved it. I followed this up with photography and became hooked on creating.

I wasn't in a good housing situation at the time, with neighbours acting in strange and unpredictable ways, which triggered my PTSD all over again. Feeling like a prisoner in my own home, and trying to find ways to distract myself from these issues, I was lead way back to fantasy and I started to create angels, fairies and mermaids from my photography. These creatures had never failed me. As an adult, they made me feel safe with them, as I did when I was a child.

My artwork is based on fairytales.

These stories of old were used for years as a moral compass, as a warning of the evil surrounding us. They also told a little girl that goodness would always prevail. During a recent battle with breast cancer, I knowingly called on my superpower to take me away from hospital treatment rooms. In my head, I was planning another story involving fantasy creatures, rather than having radiotherapy beams burn my skin. The basis of my work is 'Hope through Despair', much like my life.

So back to my superpower. Some call my superpower Dissociative Disorder (Depersonalisation) and see it as a negative. I don't. I see it as an incredible coping mechanism. It was my life saver. I'll admit I am lucky that it has been mild and only evident through times of high trauma. It has left me unable to connect emotionally most of the time, which has taken a toll on relationships. I've now accepted living with Complex PTSD, depression and anxiety, but I find that Dissociative Disorder is as effective now as it was in childhood.

These days however, it is a choice I make and is grounded and healthy. Most importantly, I have reconnected with the little girl who had the most amazing capacity to survive in a harsh world. So anyway, what's your superpower?

A self-proclaimed late bloomer and fairy-tale fanatic, Livonne is an artist and storyteller. Living with CPTSD after several traumatic, life changing events, she began writing a blog about her life, to help her heal. She was awarded Blogger of the Year 2012 followed by Most Outstanding Advocacy Blog 2013. Livonne is an award winning photography artist, specialising in fairy tales which often talk about social issues. She believes Happily Ever After is our birthright. www.Livonne.com.au

Thanks, Matthew
Bruce McMillan

I don't remember how old I was when I started thinking and feeling like that. I do remember that by the time I was in year eight in high school, I'd been thinking and feeling that way so often, and for so long, I decided I may need to talk to someone about it.

We were standing together in our cramped suburban back yard one afternoon. I can't remember what we'd been doing or talking about previously. I must have thought it was a good time, or at least as good a time as there was ever likely to be. I tried to gently phrase it as a question, anticipating the reaction.

"Do you ever feel like killing yourself?" I asked, cautiously.

As I watched, rage swept aside the initial shock, both flashing through his eyes in a millisecond. His right shoulder jerked, the arm springing back, fingers curling into a fist. Somehow, he managed to keep that fist to himself.

"Don't you ever fuckin' say that to me again!" he snarled, his voice edging toward panic.

"That's a fucking coward's way out! Don't you ever think of doing that!" His tone softening now from anger to exasperated confusion. I don't recall my reply, or even if conversation continued at all. I do remember knowing that was just another subject we wouldn't talking about around there, any time soon.

Months later, and now in year nine I decided to try again, at school this time, one sunny afternoon. We were sitting on the benches under the big gum tree, on the edge of the sports oval. Again, I don't recall what we had been talking about previously, although I have a vague sense that consternation and accusations around my recent behaviour were involved. Something must have indicated that this was a suitable opportunity. I remember how I started the conversation.

"Matthew, have you ever thought about killing yourself?"

His eyebrows knit together slightly, shocked confusion playing across his face. He blinked slowly a couple of times, considering my question.

"No! No, I haven't!" He blurted out a few moments later, his voice betraying mild panic. His eyes searched mine momentarily, before he stuttered "W-w-why, have you?"

"I think about it all the time." The honesty of my reply was surprising, even to me. Matthew stared straight through me, obviously deep in thought, digesting my reply.

"That's a very selfish thing to do," he said emphatically.

His unanticipated response baffled me somewhat.

"What do you mean? How is it selfish?" I asked.

"Well, have you thought of the people you'd leave behind?" he spluttered, exasperation creeping into his voice. "What about the person who finds your body? Have you thought about them?"

It was my turn to feel shocked and confused. No, I hadn't really considered the 'people left behind' or the 'person that found my body'. Neither of us realised it at the time, but his knee-jerk reaction is a common, though far less than ideal, response to revelations of suicidality. What I did come to realise later was that despite the panicked delivery and adolescent logic, Matthew had unwittingly revealed one of my personal protective factors against suicide.

Sometime shortly after my first birthday Dad left for work one morning and had never came home again. For seven or eight months he remained in a virtual coma, paralysed but conscious, blinking out words to my mother as she passed her index finger over an alphabet she'd written on a sheet of cardboard. She visited every day but two, the whole time he was in the hospital, and later the hospice. Mercifully, he died of encephalitis on July 13, 1967. He'd turned 40 in April.

As he lay silently fading away, she suffered serious health issues of her own. Soon after my father's death, an older sibling telephoned relatives with concerns about our mother's wellbeing. She was no longer able to get out of bed, provide for her own needs, or parent her four children. Already grief-stricken by the loss of her beloved husband, the catastrophic news had overwhelmed her. By the time she was diagnosed, the prognosis was 'terminal'. She died of cancer on November 2, 1967. She had turned 42 in September.

Immediately after our mother's death we were split into two groups of two and sent to live with friends of our parents, and with a maternal uncle and aunt. That arrangement didn't last long. Our maternal grandmother contrived to reunite us for a holiday, taking us from there back to her house, where we lived from that time on. This turn of events gave rise to a whiny refrain that was to become our organising principle, almost our family motto. Grudgingly alluding to how awful things really were, it sought simultaneously to absolve the principal adult players of any culpability: 'At least you were all together'.

My grandmother's house was the kind of place where an ever-present burden of 'gratitude' completely obliterated any possible recognition of what a counsellor later identified to me as 'physical, psychological, and spiritual abuse'. At about age six or seven, a second-cousin a couple of years my junior matter-of-factly said to me 'your Mum and Dad are dead'. That came as news to me. A few years later the next-door neighbour casually referred to a person that had 'died of cancer, like your mother', obviously assuming parental death was something we talked about. Years later, I discovered an older sibling and I had independently come to the same conclusion about our function in our grandmother's life. We were a distraction from her grief for her lost daughter. The fact her daughter had been our mother was irrelevant to her. Grief was her monopoly.

My sister, the eldest of us four siblings, was the one saving grace of life at my grandmother's house. She had sacrificed most of her adolescence bringing my middle brother and I with her when she went out with her friends. It was a prolonged and concerted effort to give us respite from the relentless barrage of threats, abuse, insults, accusations and admonishments we endured at 'home'. Matthew's response that afternoon caused me to realise I did not want to cause of any more pain in my sister's life. I did not want her to be left behind. I certainly did not want her to find my body.

By the time I talked to Matthew, substance use was already a serious issue in my life. For almost two decades alcohol and drugs would feature prominently in my life as an uncomfortably keen double-edged sword. Temporary oblivion, particularly of the alcoholic-blackout variety, afforded periodic minor relief from the intolerable revulsion of existence. The levied toll – excruciating humiliation, catastrophic self-esteem, and frequent physical assault – seemed somehow a fair exchange for the fleeting respite of wakeful unconsciousness.

Somehow my early twenties saw adult responsibility, marriage, a mortgage, and a child come flooding into my life, all financed by a succession of stop-gap, dead-end jobs. I erected a flimsy edifice of suburban 'normality' on a foundation of white-knuckled sobriety, shored-up by daily cannabis use, and reinforced with other illicit substance use, whenever the opportunity arose. After five years of alcohol use relapses, increasing in frequency and severity, it would all drain right back out again. All except the stop-gap, dead-end jobs.

The conversation with Matthew, on the edge of the oval years earlier, led me to an insufferable psychological space trapped between little desire to remain alive, and awareness of hypothetical consequences of my death by suicide. Being father of a child from an unsuccessful relationship complicated that environment considerably. Compounding concerns of distressing and aggrieving those left behind, the abysmal legacy of a parent taking their own life now also weighed frequently and heavily on my mind.

It occurred to me that if I played my cards recklessly enough, there may be a way to fold and leave the table. The distinction between 'death by misadventure' and 'suicide' on an autopsy started to look like an exit strategy. The maintenance program I'd developed – modifying Jack Daniel's consumption with heroin use – was reaching a crescendo, and a final departure acceptable to me became inevitable.

That all seems like a lifetime ago. After an admission to drug and alcohol rehab, at age 30, I remained abstinent for five-and-a-half years. A second attempt, at age 41, was 13 years ago, and I've been abstinent from drugs and alcohol ever since.

Recovery from the cumulative and compounding effects of trauma has involved a LOT of therapy, aside from drug and alcohol rehab. Years ago, I read a book by an Austrian psychoanalyst and extermination-camp survivor, who famously asked some of his patients: 'Why don't you kill yourself?' The most significant benefit of therapy and recovery for me has not been never asking that question again, but rather in finding my own meaningful and sustainable answers to it, in finding my own reasons to live.

Bruce is currently employed as a mental health peer worker by an NGO in Wollongong. Bruce is a lived-experience representative in the suicide prevention initiatives Illawarra Shoalhaven Suicide Prevention Collaborative, and Roses in the Ocean. Bruce is a member and co-facilitator of the Wollongong Hearing Voices Network group.

Cry Baby
Beate Zanner

The journey of life has been interesting when I'm known as somebody who cries easily, over nothing, or so it seems. Dealing with childhood trauma is a journey, a journey that has taken my entire life to come to terms with.

A turning point in my life was when I stopped therapy! I had been seeing a psychologist for 20 years: I needed therapy to assist when challenged by interactions with other people. Therapy helped me build the foundations, layers of skills to have faith in my abilities as a human being. Therapy certainly helped me to let out childhood pain, learn skills and reclaim feelings instead of being a 'robot of numbness'. To learn how to communicate better instead of being angry or silent – all leading to the 'hope' of a better life! I would not be where I am now without therapy.

I relied on my therapist often, and every time I had a problem, a setback, or an issue, I would either ring to talk about it, or book for an appointment to work it out further. A turning point was when I no longer wanted to work it out with therapy as it felt the same.

Something within had let me know this is me. During this time, I was unemployed due to a loss of a job and went internal by doing heaps of doona therapy. I made a big decision in not wanting to see my therapist anymore. I had realised this is me, meaning there is no cure for me. This is me in getting upset, which I find overwhelming. I do cry, easily! Sometimes this is for valid reasons to do with disappointment, disempowerment, power struggles, overwhelming emotions and feelings in not being able to speak. To speak and get my needs meet by staying and communicating. Crying is part of the human condition. I show my emotions as they say, 'on my sleeve'. Yet, there is a far greater reason for crying easily and that is childhood trauma.

Childhood trauma is part of me, so it has meant I needed to learn how to deal with myself, especially with regards to triggers. I will share a poem at this point so you can understand what it is like to be triggered. I have written a series of poems to do with triggers since working in the mental health field employed as a Peer Support Worker. Working with people with similar experiences ignited me to write poems as I realised I needed a tool to help people reclaim their life. By writing the poems it helped me reclaim my life as well through mutual and reciprocal understanding!

Trigger No. 2

Triggered! Noooo, not again!
Not feeling right……..
Thoughts of badness, and alone in the head!
This past is stuck in the present!

Thinking I need to run away! Again! (A pattern so old).
Oh! How the past is in the present!
So, in the DNA!
At any moment, the past can pop up!

Oh! My goodness!
The badness of self is present!
What do I need? What do I need? What do I need?
Support! Take a risk and share my world!

Share my world of the past
Intermixed with the present happenings.
The past that affects my present!
Allowed to be upset – now! (Really!)

Being heard, not judged, or challenged!
Instead, held, in kindness and empathy.
Whilst the shame of 'self' hovers through this interaction.
Madness prevails as I unwind to the present.

Inside – petrified! Utter Terror!
Wait, and wait for the punishment.
Thoughts and feelings of worthlessness – equals rejection!
It did not happen! The expected rejection!

Relief! Such Relief!
A chance to heal in the present!
Again, I weep with relief!
Thank you, thank you, thank you for being with me…..©

Through writing, sharing and talking about the poems with other people with similar issues, it has pushed acceptance of myself even further. More than acceptance, I met other people who have similar experiences and difficulties in their lives. Oh! What joy! Even though when I am triggered, I feel so much shame, confusion, a quagmire of past and present thoughts in my mind, I become an emotional wreck and want to run away and not be seen anymore. A trigger does not make sense when it happens. A therapist would want to know what is happening! I've learnt *talking* about it does not make sense: to be with the trigger rather than share what is happening. It is of no value when in the space of crying. A trigger can silence me, so I push people away, and opens the flood gates of the venomous inner critic of 'not good enough'. Venomous in causing problems as what comes out of my mouth is defensive as feel threatened. Or I want to 'run away due to the feelings of shame' or wanting 'to die' because I've gone to a horrible place of utter low 'self-worth' and embarrassment.

A trigger causes disconnection when you need connection in order to heal. For me the healing happens when a person can be with me, warts and all. Be it a therapist, the right friend or colleague, I think *being* with somebody is so underrated when crying or upset. Being left alone is the worst as I feel rejected! I know I find it uncomfortable with myself, but I support others when sharing pain easily. Being with me sends these messages: I want to be with you, with your pain, I don't want to fix you right now, you are okay even though upset, I've got time for you, you are a valuable person, I care for you, I love you. Even if I find this difficult, I value someone wanting to be with me, when really upset; wanting to make a cup of tea with me until I'm able to speak coherently or settled again, is helpful. My goodness, getting these messages over the years has eroded away the belief that 'I'm not a valuable person'.

Far from it, now *I am a valuable* person who wants connection and understanding in silence. Being held in a space of empathy, validated and with kindness, has helped me be with people in my perceived worst moments – when triggered. The effort has been worthwhile as I come out of the triggers quicker because other people have faith, they believe in me and love me. What great messages to receive when feeling so bad about myself – when upset by an interaction, life event or trigger, when people are confused in asking me something or giving feedback that seems so innocent.

Communicating when triggered causes so many problems with relationships, be it with family, friends or work. Having childhood trauma means I've had to learn to communicate very differently from ways I learnt during childhood. Childhood was, be seen not heard, violent interactions, and don't speak your truth as the adults in my life couldn't handle it. This caused silence, aloneness, isolation and tons of anger! As mentioned, I've learnt to find grey in between the continuum of anger and sadness. Connecting to how I am feeling means I am checking into a feeling. So freaky, as it means being with pain like sadness, or it can switch to anger which means people can be scared as it is too much. Feelings are an important guide as a human being I've learnt.

What I've missed out on was connecting to people, by staying in the conversation, processing what I heard through my body and responding accordingly. To negotiate in an adult way which is just amazing! Blows me away, as it is such a good feeling when communications go well, able to hear others, points of view, and we come out the other side intact. I realise I need to feel safe with other people to be able communicate without crying or having angry responses. Funny, sometimes I cry in relief because people have hung in there with me when interactions go well.

Power imbalances are a trigger, and I wonder if it was because I was so powerless as a child? If a manager has a certain tone of voice, looks scary, and has not engaged me in a safe manner, this is a trigger. A safe manner would be for us both to be sitting down – not me sitting and manager standing; the manager taking the time to talk to me in a kind way, not in a rush, asking questions, not telling, etc. It is hard to stay present as a part of me has gone into the rejection mode – of childhood DNA fears – in the body and mind. By been aware of what is going on for me, I can then use the many strategies I've developed over the years. If the manager is standing, I will ask them if they could sit down. It is so empowering to communicate my needs: to negotiate so I feel safe, so I can speak, so I can be an adult, so interactions can go well.

In conclusion, dealing with, and understanding what happens when I am triggered has empowered me in so many ways. I get back on the horse continually, after been upset or triggered. I remind myself that I am a human being and not a robot. I permit myself to cry, as this is what I need. The bright star that has made a difference to my life is working as a Peer Support Worker. I get to meet the most amazing people with similar experiences to me! People who have been to hell and back just like me. Being a 'cry baby' means I've got a history – nobody does anything for no reason.

Beate Zanner has been on the planet now for six decades. Beate has had many careers from stage managing in the theatre world, selling cakes, office administration, psychotherapist to now as a Peer Support Worker. Education has been key in being able to have a voice, find history and meaning for a good life! I now want to live!

Finding my way through the darkness and into the light
Candice Jade Fuller

When I was 23 years old, I went through the toughest time of my life. This is difficult for me to write about, but I hope that sharing a part of my story may have a positive impact on others, young or older, to know it's okay to not be okay and there is a way through, even if you can't see it or feel it at the time. There is always hope. We are more resilient than we know.

I have always been a very hard-working person, both academically and in sport. I feel very fortunate to have had the opportunities that I have. I grew up in a loving home with my parents and older brother, who have provided their unconditional love and support in everything I do. I've played representative sport since I was young, always pushing myself to be the best player I could be. Throughout high school, I did my best to achieve high grades and performed well in the HSC. I applied for a few different university courses. I commenced a Bachelor of Medical Science in 2008 at The University of Wollongong (UOW), with the intention to change to exercise science. I decided to stay in the medical science course and chose electives in exercise science. With a lot of 'blood, sweat and tears', I achieved my Bachelor's degree, graduating from UOW in 2010. I really enjoyed my time there, meeting great people, both students and teachers.

Towards the end of my undergraduate degree, I was deciding what I would do next. I've always had a passion for helping others and so decided to apply for a Master of Rehabilitation Counselling at the University of Sydney. I was so excited to gain entry to this course via a Commonwealth supported place. I commenced my Master's in 2011.

I'd made the decision that I really wanted to graduate with a distinction average. I was pushing myself more than ever to achieve high grades and would stress myself out so much for every test and assessment. Second year was the most challenging. We were required to complete a dissertation along with our other coursework. I also had a bad experience with an external marker which really knocked my self-confidence. To add to the pressure, I discovered I had a stress fracture in my foot from training for, and playing, netball and touch football. This was after a long and painful nine weeks of rehabilitation. I'd been misdiagnosed and hence the whole recovery process took longer. I required a cast and was on crutches for eight weeks, all while finishing up my Master's. Fortunately, my other teachers were so supportive (as well as my family and friends) and I got through second year, completing the coursework and my dissertation. I was so proud to have achieved a distinction average for my Master's! My hard work had paid off.

We were also required to complete two external placements. Via my second placement, I was lucky enough to secure my first ever full-time job as a Rehabilitation Consultant for an occupational rehabilitation provider. I was ecstatic! I would finally be starting my career – able to help people every day. My job involved supporting injured workers with a workers' compensation claim to return to work. Many workers I supported required re-training and support to find alternative employment as they couldn't return to their pre-injury roles. This was often a very difficult and emotional process for clients.

My positivity lasted for the first month. By the second month I was starting to feel so overwhelmed. I wasn't only adjusting to full-time work but working within what turned out to be a very fast-paced, high pressure industry. Some staff changes occurred, and I felt less supported, but I was determined to keep going. It was my first job, I couldn't give up. I wish I had noticed the signs earlier...

By the third month I was not coping. I couldn't switch off from work. It consumed me. It was all I could think and talk about. I couldn't sleep. I was so emotional, crying often. I did reach out to my team leader, who suggested I access the company's EAP service (Employee Assistance Program) or see my GP. Then my life came crashing down. It seemed to all happen so fast. I experienced a complete breakdown. To this day I cannot believe the impact excessive stress can have on a human being. I became so unwell. I lost the ability to articulate myself or express how I was feeling. At that time, I didn't understand what was going on for me. It was like my brain just couldn't cope anymore. Out of concern for my wellbeing, I was involuntarily admitted to a mental health unit for observation. That first night was so scary. I was given a Valium to help me feel calmer. I could not believe this was happening to me.

Over what would be the worst six weeks of my life and that of my family, I was in and out of hospital two more times. At that time, I was adamant I was a bad person and shouldn't be here anymore. I almost wasn't. Thankfully, I survived. My beautiful parents, brother, boyfriend, close family and friends were so amazing. They never gave up on me, even when I wanted to give up. To this day, I cannot thank them enough for their unconditional love and support.

Something very profound happened in hospital which has stuck with me. Really struggling one day, I asked my psychiatrist, "what is wrong with me?" to which he replied, "there is nothing wrong with you, you are just dealing with what has happened." This was so powerful for me in my early stages of recovery. It helped me accept that this wasn't my fault.

That it was okay, however, bad things can happen in life. After my final discharge from hospital I was linked with the most amazing psychologist. I can't thank her enough for helping me process the traumatic memories, thoughts, feelings and experiences I had. She helped me make sense of it all and slowly build myself back up over many years, along with my family and close friends.

There were many other important factors in my long-term recovery. On the 29th November 2013, I attended my graduation for my Master's degree, just two months after being so unwell and thinking my life was over. It was the greatest day.

2014 was a big year. I trialled and was selected in a premier league women's team for touch football (my favourite sport) which was huge for me, and since then have loved being a part of such an awesome team. I found volunteer work within mental health and I started studying again. I had always considered completing my fitness courses and working as a Fitness Instructor one day. I'm extremely proud to have achieved my Certificate III and IV in Fitness, not that long after being discharged from hospital. I started working as a Fitness Instructor that same year and absolutely loved it (and still do). I'm also proud to have not given up on my passion for counselling work. I enrolled in a Diploma of Counselling on a full-time study load in 2015, while working part-time in the fitness industry and I worked for six months as a youth worker. I completed my Diploma in 2017. That same year, I finally secured a paid job in the mental health field after applying a total of five times, starting back in 2014.

Now, I also work as a Mental Health Peer Support Worker, working with a great team to support people with their physical health and wellbeing as well as their mental health recovery. I utilise my lived experience knowledge to inspire others and create hope that they too can achieve their personal recovery goals, whatever they may be. Personal recovery is not easy. It might sound very cliché, but it is a journey and has its ups and downs.

In 2016, I went through another tough time with my mental health. Not to the extent of my 2013 experiences but it was still a really hard time. I reached out to my support network and with their support, some time and my own resilience, I made it through again. Over the past few years, I've also had to be resilient with my physical health. I've ruptured the anterior cruciate ligaments (ACL) in both my knees within 17 months of each other playing my favourite sport, touch football. It was devastating. I've had two knee reconstruction surgeries and had to go through two lengthy rehabilitation processes.

Reflecting on it all, I'm so proud of myself. I am doing very well. I am so grateful to be alive. Don't get me wrong, I still have some hard days, but I am committed to staying well, both physically and mentally. I am so fortunate to have my beautiful family and close friends who have been by my side throughout it all, my psychologist, and the ability to pursue different areas of work and study that I'm so passionate about. I'm still interested in counselling work and hope to pursue it again in the future, but for right now I'm grateful to be where I am, while always seeking to be the best person I can be. I am enough!

I hope that this snippet of my story can help educate and inspire others (particularly young people) about coping with mental health challenges and that no matter how bad you feel at a certain point, there is always a way to work through it. I want to encourage anyone who might be struggling at the moment to reach out, there is support out there and you too can find your way through.

Candice is a Peer Support Worker and member of the physical health team at a community mental health service. She is also a Registered Group Exercise Instructor and Personal Trainer with Fitness Australia. Candice has achieved a Bachelor of Medical Science, Master of Rehabilitation Counselling, Certificate III and IV in Fitness, Diploma of Counselling and Certificate IV in Mental Health Peer Work. She is passionate about helping others, particularly with their health, fitness and wellbeing.

Living with Borderline
Paul Miners

"Mental illness"! "Mental illness"! "Mental illness"! You may as well be saying the 'f' word. It doesn't matter how many times you say it, how you say it, how loud you say it or what context you put it in. They are two words that come with a stigma attached.

I have lost friends, lost jobs, and have been made to feel isolated because of these two words. Yes I suffer from mental illness. I didn't ask for it nor did I want it, but I have it and have had to learn to live with it. I didn't go to the doctors and say, "hey I want to be different, give me a cool illness, one where I can feel good one day and bad the next...I want to feel so bad that I will wish that I was never born, so bad that one day I will even try to end my existence".

The stigma that comes with mental ill-health is the reason I haven't shared my story until today. Why am I sharing my story you ask? Because I want others to understand. I want the stigma to disappear. I want to help others, who live or have lived, a life like mine.

I have always been the type of person who over analyses and over exaggerates everything. What is small to someone else is quite often very large and very real to me. I am a kind-hearted person, empathetic to others and will run from and avoid confrontation at all costs.

I left school at the end of year 10 to do an apprenticeship as a signwriter. It was a high paying job which required great skill. Then in the 90s computers came along, took away the skill and lowered the wages. My job title changed from a tradesman signwriter to a graphic designer within the sign industry which earned a very low wage.

I was married at the young age of 21 (I am 48 now) and had a child. The marriage didn't last long and when my son was three months old my ex-wife went back to a previous boyfriend and made it very hard for me to see my son. In 2002, I remarried and now have three fantastic teenage children.

My story starts back in 2013. My wife and I had committed to a rather large mortgage in 2007, and when the interest rates went sky high, we never really got back on our feet financially after our purchase. In 2013, our finances got so bad that my wife and I had a rather large disagreement over the phone, which in my head, was a lot larger than it really was.

The phone conversation occurred in the morning prior to work. By the time it got to lunch time, I was experiencing emotions that I had never experienced before and no matter how much I tried to move forward from these emotions, I was slipping deeper and deeper into severe depression. It went from a little stressed about finances in the morning, to thinking I was a bad father, a bad provider and wanting to end my life. I left work without telling anyone, went into the bush and had my first attempt on my life.

The attempt didn't go as planned and I was able to call a psychologist who I had only started seeing three weeks prior. She managed to talk me out of the bush, to go to a hospital. That day I admitted myself into a private mental health hospital and spent three weeks there.

When I left hospital, things just went back to how they were – except I was treated a little differently. People were tip-toeing around me in case they upset me. Some tried to help and others avoided me. My time in hospital hadn't really helped and it wasn't long before the severe depression started to take over again. I am not sure what the trigger was this time but again I ran from home and tried to take my life. This time it wasn't a serious attempt but enough to end up back in the private mental health hospital. But this time it was different. My depression went from bad to worse. You wouldn't think it could get any worse, but it did.

It didn't matter how many anti-depressants I took, how many times I talked to a Psychologist or how many group classes I took, I wasn't getting any better. I saw for the first time how it was affecting my wife and children. That was enough to take me into an even deeper state of depression. I left the hospital and again tried to take my life. I ended up in the PECC unit (Psychiatric Emergency Care Centre) of my local hospital and was scheduled. I couldn't leave on my own will.

After two weeks I was allowed back to the private hospital, but I was no better. I had very low self-esteem and hated who I had become. I decided that I was not a good provider, husband or father and didn't deserve what I had. I thought it would be better for my wife and kids if I end the marriage, move out and live on my own. I even tried to make the marriage look bad so that I could find that way out.

After three months in hospital, with a few visits to the PECC unit, I went boarding with a patient I had met in hospital. That was not a good move for someone with my condition. It very quickly went from a boarder to something else. This just made my state of mind worse. Not only was I not good enough for my family but I was making myself feel worse by what I was doing. I would sit outside and smoke a packet of cigarettes thinking and stressing about what I had done to my wife and kids. I missed them so much. I had destroyed their lives with my depression. I had another couple of visits to hospital via ambulance whilst living in this situation.

After a year, I moved out into a flatting situation to try and make a life for myself on my own and fight my mental illness. I was OK for a while and started feeling better and then ended up in a volatile relationship with an alcoholic. A number of things went wrong in this situation. Severe depression started creeping back in again. One day when I had my kids over for a visit, this person got quite drunk and was nasty to my kids and to myself. This was the last straw for me. I had destroyed my life and the lives of my kids and wife.

I put my kids in the car and proceeded to take them home. The drive took an hour, giving me time to plan my exit from a world that I felt I didn't belong in. I had attempts on my life prior and with the failures I seemed to get better at perfecting it. I won't share what I did – let's just say that I was found unconscious by an off duty police officer who wasn't even supposed to be in the area. I was lucky (unlucky in my mind) to be alive. I was taken to hospital by ambulance.

Following my stay in emergency, and the short stay part of the hospital, I was scheduled into my local public hospital in the Mental Health unit. It was whilst in the mental health unit that my wife came to help me. She bought me clothes and when released from hospital, offered a place for me to stay in the bottom of her house, while I was recovering. It felt bad for a long time.

I felt I didn't deserve it. How could I accept this? How could she forgive me?

I couldn't even forgive myself. It was these thoughts and negative thinking that made me run off one more time. I was on the news, the internet and in the papers as a missing person. Whilst missing, I was sleeping on the beach. This gave me time to do some soul searching. I fought my way out of a depressed state and went to the local mental health community centre. I saw people who helped me. They listened and understood. They didn't judge.

I was previously diagnosed with Bipolar Disorder, and put on Lithium. I had the extreme lows but definitely not the extreme highs. However, on this occasion, a fantastic psychiatrist changed my diagnosis to Borderline Personality Disorder. There are similar characteristics to Bipolar but there was a slightly different approach to treatment.

People from the centre would come and see me at my home, and were there whenever I needed to talk. They enrolled me in a DBT (Dialectical Behaviour Therapy) group which was fantastic. I had done groups before but this time I was ready to try. DBT was confronting, it bought up things from my younger days that I had suppressed. Things that would tip anyone over the edge. Rape, bullying and the list goes on.

I am back with my family and slowly working through things. I am back in the work force, learning to deal with life's stresses in other ways. I still have days/weeks of depression and occasional negative thoughts but have learnt to fight my way through the best I can.

For people who don't understand the severity of severe depression, I would describe it as being stuck in a dark deep hole with no way out: the hole just keeps getting deeper and deeper. Some people help you dig that hole without even realising they are holding a shovel.

The worst thing someone can do is tell you to just get over it, be strong, do some exercise, and I feel like I have to walk on egg shells around you.

If I could do all these things, don't you think I would?

For a number of years suicide was my security blanket. If I hit rock bottom with my depression, I would try to take my life. Eventually I learnt to change my security blanket from suicide to focusing on some of the techniques I had learnt in DBT. Having people around who understand mental illness helps more than anything. People who don't judge, don't get angry with you, who understand who you are and what you are going through.

I have had to leave out a number of other terrible things that have happened along the way but hopefully this gives an insight to how mental illness can consume your life and how a few simple things can make things a lot better.

Paul is an international award-winning artist who has a strong commitment to sharing his lived experience as a way of helping others suffering at the hands of mental illness. Paul hopes to help reduce the stigma of mental illness and suicide in Australia. In his spare time, he loves to paint, go on stand-up paddle boarding adventures and play tennis with his children. Paul immigrated to Australia from New Zealand in 1999.

Lion girl
Zoe Glen Norman

She needs to be tamed. They throw everything they've got at her: therapy, medication. They try to pin her down with words. Yet nothing can dull the force that moves her in undefinable ways. A force as stoppable as a tsunami. She longs to free herself. To run. To smash. To climb. Life is her playground. Death is her shadow. And the one who calms the beast will be her eternal master.

~*~

It's hard to tell where it all began, just as it's hard to tell where a ball of string begins. But by the time I was twenty, my life was one tangled mess. I was a shell of my former self, an inverted version where the world around me was now light, and I was black. I was nocturnal. I couldn't deal with anything. I no longer dived headfirst into new adventures but approached the world with hesitation. The one thing I loved the most – company – I now hated. I had internalised my enormous energy and emotions; they clawed at my insides, desperate for expression. And I spent my days lost in cyberspace instead of the real world. Suddenly I realised I was a prisoner. A prisoner inside my own mind. While I had just survived twelve years of bullying and social exile, the loneliness that struck me after I graduated felt so much worse. My will to live flipped into a will to death; suicide became my only hope.

~*~

I was fifteen when I first realised my mind was unravelling. I had just moved to my second college after a nightmare year at my first. A year that got progressively worse, like a crescendo which never resolves. I needed a fresh start, and was sent to a small Christian college on the other side of the hill. I already had a friend there, Kayla, who used to live a few doors down from me when I was little. The school was also spacious, with a lake and open green plains stretching into the horizon; plenty of room to get away from people.

"You will shine here," my father told me.

Before I knew it, I was cloaked in a straight, no-nonsense navy blazer over the top of Kayla's old checkered dress. I smelt of somebody else's perfume, but as much as I wished I was a new person, my past continued to haunt me.

My first experience of mental illness felt like being stuck on stage before a scathing audience. I remember passing a group of students on the lawn. They were laughing, and I was convinced it was me they were laughing at.

At parties, I would just sit on the couch stiff and lifeless as Kayla and her friends spun and swirled before me.

"Come dance," Kayla would insist, trying to pull me up from the couch.

All I wanted was to disappear into the shadows. Eventually I could no longer contain the monster within. The small room, full of noise and people, felt like a gas chamber. I had to get out. Suddenly I found myself getting up, as though controlled by invisible strings, and charging for the nearest exit. I wrenched the sliding door open and stepped into the patio, gasping for solitude like an asthmatic gasps for air. There was a basketball there and I began kicking it against the wall… anything to distract me.

I never knew what to do with party invites from that day onwards. My brain just couldn't handle them. Nor could it handle the pain of not being invited. I worried I would upset the person if I turned down their invite, so agreed to come. I would then pull out last minute, making up a phony excuse, such as my parents wouldn't drive me. But I just didn't seem to win, whatever I did.

"Any parent would take their daughter to a party if their daughter really wanted to go," Kayla's friend grilled me the next day.

"If you didn't want to go, you could have just said from the start. Our friend was looking forward to seeing you, and I saw the disappointment in her face when you told her you weren't coming anymore."

After giving me the guilt trip, she dredged up her own party from our memory banks.

"You practically walked out of my party," she accused.

I had similar experiences at school camps, breaking down at breakfast time, or when people ran through the dormitories playfully chasing each other with pillows. I eventually left this school also, but my social anxiety stayed with me. I didn't have much success making friends at my final college. In the end I resigned to my aloneness. I spent recess and lunchtime in the library with my textbooks. This meant that I often skipped meals; I wasn't allowed to eat in the library and, buoying around outside on my own eating, I was hyper-aware of my every move: the way I stood like a moron, stroppy and aimless. The motion of my mouth as I bit and chew my food. The space I took up.

My anxiety spread to all areas of my life. I put enormous pressure on myself to achieve, studying at recess and lunchtime, on school excursions, on the bus, and the minute I got home. It was during my final two years of school I got a glimpse of the obsessive compulsive beast in me, a force that refuses to be stopped. Sometimes I broke under the pressure, tears streaming down my face in the middle of tests. My heart raced and I couldn't remember how to answer the questions despite studying so hard. In one maths test I got up part way through and, trembling, handed my blank paper to the teacher before walking out. But I continued to push on, and, somehow, ended up school dux. I was told, with grades like mine, I could do anything and be anyone I wanted to be. I'm not so sure. I think the school would be shocked where I've ended up.

~*~

Over the years there have been a few people who have taken an interest in me and shown me kindness. These people have become saints in my eyes. Lights in a world of darkness. Personal saviours. But this has only paved the way for a whole new set of problems. The trajectory goes as follows: I let these people in, I believe my happy ending has arrived, they become my everything, I find myself strapped into a cosmic rollercoaster which takes me as high as the stars then straight to the ocean floor when this person leaves. It's the worst pain I have felt in my life. It would be kinder to die than go through this, and indeed I am left begging for death to take me.

My first experience of this was with a teacher during my final years of school. She was the only one who asked me if I was ok. It was just three simple words, but it meant the world to me. I always said I was fine, that I liked being alone. But secretly I longed to tell her everything. When I heard she was leaving the school, I fell into the deepest of depressions. As soon as I got home that day I went straight to bed and didn't get up. I kept the curtains drawn and buried my face into my pillow. The tears were no longer flowing properly so the searing pain remained trapped inside. My family didn't know what was wrong with me. I didn't even know what was wrong with me, I just wanted to die. My only grace was that I got this teacher's email address. But unfortunately it was only a taste of what was coming. The next person this happened with, was a counsellor I saw at university, my very first therapist. I have learnt that the pain of finding love and then losing it is worse than the pain of not being loved at all. We realise how life could be, should be, and then it is taken away from us. Losing my counsellor tipped me into a depression I'm still trying to climb out of to this day.

My collection of diagnoses has grown substantially over the last many years. Anxiety turned into depression which turned into personality disorders, an eating disorder, a sleep disorder, ADD, autism, prodrome psychosis. I tried several medications which did nothing to control the ravaging beast inside me. I started to wonder if the beast was actually outside of me. I lost all sense of safety in the world, terrified of the invisible, silent pollution from phone towers, satellites and 'smart' meters. Major depression has now been changed to schizoaffective, autism has been scrapped, and prodrome psychosis has been changed to psychosis. It seems like the professionals can't even agree with each other, and just when they think they have it pinned, it changes form. But I suspect that this lion, deep down, is not that different from us all. This lion just wants to live its stolen youth. This lion just wants to break free.

And I suspect she doesn't need a whiz-bang therapy or breakthrough drug so much, but something we all need: love.

"Love one another and you will be happy," wrote Leunig. "It's as simple and as difficult as that."[1]

Zoe Glen-Norman is an emerging writer from Melbourne. In her spare time, which she has plenty of due to her de-railed life, she "overdoses" on music, the computer and Netflix, smacks shuttlecocks, and fantasises about running away to the country. Somewhere along the way she picked up a degree in psychology. Zoe's website is: www.zonkyzoe.com

1 Michael Leunig, Australian cartoonist, writer, painter, philosopher and poet.

Seduction of Business: the Early Days
Douglas Holmes

Douglas's journey started back in 1949 in a small country town on the Mid North Coast of NSW called Bellingen. He attended the Bellingen Catholic primary school in 1955 and had from what he remembers a pretty happy childhood.

In January 1961, I remember being out on the farm, during the Xmas holidays, milking the cows and doing chores. I arrived home excited about starting at Bellingen Public High School. Unfortunately, this dream did not happen due to dysfunction in our family: mum decided to withdraw from the violence she was subjected to – on a regular basis – when dad lost his pay in the poker machines.

The family, minus dad, ended up in a house in Valla. Without funds for the bus to the high school in Macksville, the decision was made to send me to Valla Public Primary school, where I repeated sixth class.

Over the next the next four years the family (minus dad) moved around a lot, mainly to get away from dad's behaviour, as his drinking and gambling were progressing.

In 1965 I applied to join the Navy and in October I turned up in York Street, Sydney, for the enrolment process. Unfortunately, my application for my dream job was turned down. I came back to Newcastle with a chip on my shoulder that over time turned into telegraph poles. The words of the naval recruitment officer were ringing in my ears, "Mr Holmes, why did you want to join the navy?" I replied, "Early retirement, see the world, and have a girl in every port".

"Well Holmes", continued the naval recruitment officer, "we have some bad news for you. Your test shows that you will develop some problems. Go home and get some help". In 1965 there was not the assistance that a lot of us take for granted today, so I stumbled along. In 1991, whilst living on the South Coast of NSW, near Batemans Bay, I hit the wall with what was described as a nervous breakdown.

There were no hospital beds vacant and I was managed in the community. I was referred to the Black Dog Institute at Prince Henry Hospital in Malabar: there I learned about Bipolar Affective Disorder and the wonder drug Lithium that would fix the 'chemical imbalance'. Lithium was discovered in the same year I was born. I decided to leave Batemans Bay and returned to Newcastle in 1992.

In Newcastle, I went onto the Sickness Benefit: I joined the mental illness psychosocial merry-go-round, ending up in a Hunter Health group home in Cardiff. In 1994, I received a Disability Support Pension.

Fortunately, the Australian Government started the National Mental Health Strategy, and the First (five-year) National Mental Health Plan. Hunter Health was including consumers and carers to improve mental health services across the Hunter.

I got involved. Besides having a purpose and a routine, there were other benefits. I got support to attend interesting meetings and events including the opportunity to attend the 1996 Brisbane TheMHS Conference, with an all-expenses paid trip to Brisbane to attend the TheMHS Consumer

Day, with three other consumers from Newcastle, to see what was happening in other places across Australia, with participation.

I heard Patricia Deegan use her own lived experience when she delivered the keynote address titled: *The sea rose: Recovering from mental illness*[1], and this was significant. As she talked about how she felt when she was given her diagnosis at 18, having her dreams taken away, it took me back to those times in my life when similar things had happened in my journey: not going onto high school with a group of friends that I had grown up with, and being told at 16 to go home and get some help, when there was no help available.

Another keynote speaker was Charles Rapp who talked about the Strengths Model, widely used in Kansas, and the need for consumers to be allowed to go through their 'woodshed' period to work out what they wanted to do with the rest of their life.

The term 'woodshed' relates to when a person is learning to play the saxophone: he or she is often put out in the woodshed to practice. I understood this to mean that the timeout I was having on the Disability Support Pension would allow me to formulate a plan to change the way mental health services were delivered in Australia, and what part I wanted to play in those changes.

I was inspired to change mental health services so that other consumers would have a better recovery journey than I and my family had in the previous 36 years.

I had an awakening – that all that was wrong for me was that my dreams

---

1 Deegan, P.E. (1996). *The sea rose: Recovering from mental illness. There's a Person in Here: Contemporary themes in mental health services*, The Mental Health Services Conference Inc. of Australia and New Zealand: Ian Liddell Pty Limited, p. xvi–xxiv.

had been crushed – and I needed to find other ways to reawaken those dreams.

In 1998, I came off Lithium, and remain on course to achieve my dreams.

With these two new bits of knowledge, I returned to Newcastle and set out on a new course of action that involved moving to Sydney. I still remember the concern most people had when I announced my plan.

Another interesting thing happened. In 1996, Professor Beverley Raphael, the Director of the NSW Centre for Mental Health, gave the NSW Consumer Advisory Group Mental Health Inc. (NSW CAG) money to run a forum to look at what consumers and carers wanted services to look like twenty years on, in 2016.

A report, *From Consumer to Citizen*[2], was released with 10 issues that were workshopped.

The 10 issues were:
1.   Standards
2.   Training Needs
3.   Consumer Positions and Networks
4.   Independent Assessment of Services
5.   Guidelines/Payments
6.   Partnerships
7.   Clarification of Government Responsibility
8.   Paid Advocacy
9.   Respite
10.   Consumers from Non-English Speaking Background, Ageing, Aboriginal and Torres Strait Islanders, Gay and Lesbian Consumers, Multiple Disabilities and other groups.

---

2 *NSW Consumer Advisory Group (1996). From Consumer to Citizen, NSW Consumer Advisory Group, Rozelle. https://auspwn.files. wordpress.com/2014/05/from-consumer-to-citizen-v-1-original-230106.pdf*

I was a member of NSW CAG from 1997 – 2000; a founding member of the Australian Mental Health Consumer Network from 1997; and I was NSW CAG's Executive Officer from 2000 – 2006. My goal was to embed consumer participation at the core of mental health services in NSW.

From 2006 – 2017, I was fortunate to work with staff at St Vincent's Hospital, as the Mental Health Consumer Participation Officer, to put the policies we worked on into action.

I was awarded the TheMHS Exceptional Achievement Award, in 2014. The award states: "The awards represent an acknowledgement of an exceptional contribution, the results of which will flow on to enhance the mental health and wellbeing of all."

On my certificate, TheMHS included the following words: "This award is for recognition of unswerving dedication to the betterment of services to support consumer wellbeing; for extraordinary determination to ask questions and seek out answers; for outstanding expertise, freely given, with a 'can do' attitude whether it be for national policy or a local art group."

In 2018, I was awarded the Medal of the Order of Australia in the General Division for services to the Community.

My only regret is that NSW has not followed through with an audit of the 10 issues that consumers and carers identified in the *From Consumer to Citizen* report.

Douglas is the Founder and Patron of MH-worX.com. Douglas became a member of the NSW Consumer Advisory Group Mental Health Inc. (NSW CAG) from 1997 to 2000, and a founding member of the Australian Mental Health Consumer Network from 1997. He became the NSW CAG's Executive Officer from 2000 till 2006. Douglas retired from St Vincent's as the Consumer Participation Officer in 2017.

Abnormal: Normality is a Falsehood
Hannah Gabrielle

They told me to stop.
Stop what? I said.
Stop creating.
The very essence of who I am, the very detriment to my wellbeing.
My passion pushed to one side, made a separate entity, separate from me.
Creativity? No, it is my enemy.
Now medicated to a lifeless existence, creativity squeezed right out of me.
This is how I will be.

///

Bipolar.
It's a complex disorder.
Often labelled manic-depression.
They think the diagnosis means you're moody. But no, it's a sustained
high, or sustained low.
The highs can last weeks.

Mania is founded in the spinning overwhelm with every touch, sound,
light, and emotion.
The highs are euphoric. You are increasingly aroused; on top of the world.
You are at your happiest – but they call you too happy.
Everything that goes up must come down.

The anxiety you experience feels like you're drowning,
except you can see everyone around you breathing
It's like trying to breathe when you're covered in tar.
You can't control it, you feel like it controls you.
It's not made up just to get attention. Who would want to live like this.
It's fear,
It's emptiness,
It's numbness,
It's shame.

Beyond the anxiety, psychosis exists.
It lies in the morning mist over your inhibitions; you can't see clearly.
You sometimes imagine things that aren't real.
You're easily agitated. You're fearful.
You might think people are following you.
You might think demons will conquer you.

You feel threatened, yet you think you can take on the world.
You are a dreamer, but they call you too ambitious.
You are too vocal; too theatrical. Is that even a thing?
The illness is mistaken for the creativity that explodes from your being.

The lows however, bring depression. You lose perspective.
The despair you feel is like a black fog; you just can't see through it.
You feel like a ghost – not a part of the real world.
A total loss of who you are
The belief that you don't matter

Treatment is being told that you must cease your creativity.
Forced low stimulus. Restrained expression.
You walk a tightrope, balancing the joys and difficulties of life stressors.
You find yourself in a resulting squirm for autonomy and self-expression.
Previously you were flying.
Now have a set of shackles on your arms and legs, you are tied down.
In treatment, everyone's critiquing your condition.
It feels like you're walking down a red carpet, and you're naked.

One day you will learn the art of the giraffe;
to have your head in the clouds
but your feet on the ground.

*This poetry titled, Abnormal: Normality is a Falsehood, was written
in collaboration with mental health survivors, for a performance
with Yellow Wheel Dance Company in 2018. Hannah is an artist and
graduating psychology and dance student from Deakin University, who
is pursuing ongoing research into the intersection of dance and mental
health.*

Through the Generations: A Mother's journey towards open communication
Siobhan T – A Mum in her 50s

The lack of emotional connection I experienced as a child has had a powerful, negative influence on my life and on my children. I hope and pray that my family's inability to share difficulties is now being broken down and there will be a growing trust and openness. I am sure that openness will lead to greater understanding, to forgiveness and to healthier relationships in the next generation. If issues are not addressed serious dysfunction can be handed down through generations.

There were too many 'no go' areas in my family when I was growing up. There were many questions I couldn't ask, and when I did ask, they were shut down. There were emotions such as anger and disappointment that were unacceptable for me to express.

And this legacy had an impact on my children. There were too many things I felt unable to talk about: too many secrets that affected my children when they were growing up.

When I was growing up, I learned to keep any distressing feeling (frustration, anger, disappointment, hurt, confusion, fear) inside. When I shared any of these feelings with my Mum, the result was rejection, abandonment. An invisible wall, like a castle wall, would erupt from the ground. My Mum's face would freeze – she couldn't cope, she froze, she panicked and was emotionally out of there. I would be alone, worse off... so I learned not to talk about anything difficult.

This meant I also 'shut-down' these unacceptable emotions. They got buried 'under the carpet' before they even surfaced. Unacceptable. No place for these feelings because I want to stay connected. Don't go there. Ever. I learned it hard. And I learned it strong. I learned to only speak about positives.

The problem is that 'under the carpet', these emotions twist and turn and change into something else. They are part of life. There is peril in ignoring them. In my life, they turned to depression and despair. I spoke positives but my thoughts were filled with negative self-criticism.

Some other factors that affected my life negatively were:

- my high expectations (impossible ones, upon reflection now);

- my belief that my role was to keep everyone happy;

- no love for myself, no boundaries;

- my husband demanding and needing to be 'right'. He didn't know how to encourage or apologise. Blame, lectures about shortcomings, and I felt absolutely inadequate and a failure;

- moving between four different states in Australia when my husband graduated from university and when he changed jobs. I was isolated from long term friends and family. I left my job in Melbourne and there were no similar opportunities in the country towns we then moved to.

All these factors combined as a 'perfect storm' for a downward spiral. It happened. Big time. I experienced depression from when my son and daughter were two and four years old. The darkness inside me became so strong that I believed I was causing damage just by being with people. I overdosed. I survived and spent some long periods in a private clinic and in the mental health wards of public hospitals. I came back home each time and acted like nothing had happened. I didn't know how to talk about it.

But my kids were affected, and they were worried. They were traumatised by what happened, surrounded by secrets and our 'no-go' areas. Now they are in their 20s and have said to me "Mum: you got counselling. Dad got counselling. How come we kids didn't get counselling?" Good question.* In twenty years of professional counselling, no counsellor ever discussed how I could talk with my kids about what I was going through! No-one even mentioned it.

Hello!!

Kids are people too!! My distress as a parent affected them greatly.

Four sentences may have been enough: "I am sorry that I have been away from home. I missed you. If you want to ask me something – please ask me anytime. I might need some time to think, but I will get back to you."

A brief acknowledgement would have at least reduced the secrets, though it would still have been a terribly difficult time for us all.

The silence and lack of support for my kids made it worse. They had no-one to ask because it was a 'no go' zone. No trust. Secrets. Anger. Doubt. Worry. Chronic stress. What is going on with Mum? What is real? What is true?

My Recovery Journey

My journey towards recovery began when I was enrolled in weekly group therapy courses as an out-patient. (My 'children' were 18 and 20 years of age by this time.) I was desperate. I would try anything. I had already undergone electroconvulsive therapy (ECT) quite a few times. I was prescribed a plethora of anti-depressants over many years. Many hours of counselling. Many counsellors.

I started attending group therapy when I was at my lowest ebb ever. No hope. But I followed the instructions I was given. Obedient and compliant (as usual) I attended a two-hour session each week with two facilitators and about eight other participants.

'Dealing with Depression', my first group ... A glimmer of light.

Other Groups. 'Healthy Relationships', 'Managing Emotions', 'Assertiveness' and 'Mindfulness'.

Looking forward to the classes... starting to talk about myself. Learning about the internal battles other lovely people are facing.

Dialectical Behaviour Therapy (DBT). Schema Therapy. Now this is getting deep!!! Some huge 'aha' moments! New perspectives. A realisation that all emotions have a purpose...starting to be able to reflect on difficult emotions... using WISE MIND (from DBT) to finally acknowledge and be aware of my anger and fear. I could now evaluate things and choose what to do in response to my difficult emotions.

Assertiveness to say what I think is fair, what I think is happening, what I want... even to (gently) confront!! WOW! What a change is happening!

Realising that I am ONLY responsible for my own happiness. I want to be kind to others. but I AM NOT RESPONSIBLE FOR HOW THEY FEEL. They have that responsibility.

FREEDOM!!! ADEQUACY!!! BLESSED RELIEF!!! BURDENS LIFTED!!!

Jump forward two years... the only group therapy course I haven't done is the one about 'Managing Anxiety'. While doing this course... I realise that I am not learning much in this group... maybe I am ready for 'graduating' from group therapy... what next?

I found that there are other supportive groups – like the Western Australian Association for Mental Health (WAAMH), Drop the Disorder, and Consumers of Mental Health WA (COMHWA). I started doing my own reading, doing other courses about mental health, attending conferences, some paid work as a consumer representative and as a 'lived experience educator'.

I am empowered and want to help others realise their strengths, to learn new skills and perspectives that can help them 'climb out' from whatever pit of mental distress they are experiencing.

I know we are all different, but I think the current mental 'health' system is too medicalised. I think it doesn't listen. I think it is disempowering to many people and causing further damage. We have the answers to our own healing within us. We just need help to develop our strengths and new perspectives and skills. We need support while practicing these new skills.

And the news about my family? Difficulties. My husband and I have separated. Our adult children are very angry with us for the deception and secrets that were part of our family for so many years.

I am gradually working through things with my kids.

The joy and benefits of being able to talk about my emotions are wonderful and, with practice, I am gaining wisdom in how much to share in varying situations.

I am empowered and want to make a difference for others experiencing mental distress and their children. I am so excited that I have been able to contribute to this wonderful collaborative book!

I hope you can accept yourself 'warts and all', have realistic expectations, care for yourself and (sustainably) care for others! I hope my story will help give you courage to look at what is happening in your life. And even greater courage to talk about some deep things and to apologise for the mistakes that you make. (Yes, we all make mistakes!). I believe that talking openly enables healing, growth, forgiveness, restoration and authentic, caring relationships. And healthy relationships are vital for living well!!

Suggestion for Medicare: when a parent has a Mental Health Care Plan, the children also need free access to see an empathetic therapist, who has deep listening skills. (headspace, which provides Australia-wide services, ages 12 – 25 is a start.)

**Please note: I love my Mum and know that she loves me and did the best job she could. I have forgiven my Mum for the emotional gaps that* *have affected me. I know my Mum was stuck just as I got stuck. I am so very thankful for the groups that helped enable me to think differently and communicate more openly. My Mum's love language is 'acts of service'. She doesn't usually talk about the past at all. I am hoping to have the courage to start (very gently) asking her some questions about when my sisters and I were on the farm growing up. I really hope to gradually get to know her more (without causing those castle walls to rise)! Start with the good times. Little steps!*

Siobhan T is going well now after suffering Major Depression for many years. The transformation for Siobhan came through insights and skills gained by attending weekly Group Therapy for two years. Siobhan believes that the most significant factors in overcoming her depression have been learning to: acknowledge ALL emotions (including anger), talk openly about ALL her feelings and experiences, set personal boundaries, be kind to herself, be assertive and to have achievable expectations.

Seeds
MD Rasel Khandokar Kasmer

What I am going to discuss with you now is very interesting, and a little bit scary for me as everything is a bit scary for me at the beginning, like talking to the customers, or using a knife for chopping up vegetables. But what I am going to talk about is a bit more serious. But if I can muster this, I think I can gain inner peace in a deeper way. I can be closer to Allah as a Muslim believes. I can find more answers as to who I am, why I am here. This world. Good and bad. Negative and positive. Negative energy and positive energy that's what I am talking about. I was in this spiritual state before, but I was also mentally very unwell, and I did not know how to look after my mental health. So, I could not find these answers. But I have mental support now. I will check my reality with a psychologist and, if you want, you can do this with your family or friends before we go further.

I am listening to this famous (audio) book 'The Power of Now' by Eckhart Tolle. I am half- way through that book but I cannot wait to stir things a little bit now. My main focus will be energy. No, no... not the energy we use for lighting our rooms or to run a car or anything of this sort, but the energy in the human body. The energy and power of the human mind. Do not think me crazy yet, but I also think about the energy and power of human heart. I think I am talking about spirituality. Spiritual energy. Can you feel it?

First of all, I would like to mix physics with spirituality. Newton says energy can neither be created nor destroyed, rather it can only be transformed or transferred from one from to another. Yeah, Newton was talking about energy and trains, but I think I am talking about more valuable energy; the energy of the heart and brain. But I think we can use the same theory for spiritual energy. Before I go further I will say it is very easy to balance negative energy and positive energy by following the Quran or true monotheism. Because who created us knows better than what we think or know, about the energy of the brain or heart. And Quran is Allah's word. (Go to Google or YouTube to find why you will believe Quran is Allah's word.)

Now, I want to explore spirituality and mental health. When I was suffering from high anxiety and depression, I was thinking my spiritualty could help me get rid of my disease. I know it is never too late… but I think it was too late. But it was also only the beginning of a new straight path. I was taking medication for high anxiety and depression, as well as practicing my spiritual beliefs in order to fight my disease. But now I think my brain and heart realised there was too much negative energy all around me at that time, and for many environmental reasons it could no longer be balanced, or there was universal negative energy. Can you see the energy we are all using? Energy of the universe.

If you are a psychiatrist you do hard work thinking… "what can I do to balance the chemicals in the brain?" So we found such chemicals for now – chemicals to create a negative energy or positive energy. Universal negative energy – power, fighting, dominating natures, hatred, guilt, worry, anxiety, depression, schizophrenia, and so on from negative energy. For the millions of people who lost their lives in world wars. Can you see that universal negative energy is building up again through negative information or negative data? What is the anti-psychotic medication for that? Please look at the positives not negatives. Please look at the similarities not differences.

As I said when I was trying to find answer in relation to my spirituality and my mental illness, it was making me paranoid, fearful, anxious, guilty, addicted, a 'no-trust-in-anybody' type feeling – even though I was a practicing Muslim. At the time, this had a lot of bad impacts. But because I then started practicing my spiritual beliefs, I just found everything to be easy. I don't know, I just said 'it could be worse' to myself, I just said He who created me with love will solve all my problems, I do not have to worry about the future (even though I had lots of guilt). I said to myself Allah will forgive me of my past, all I am appreciating is my present. This was tough but enjoyable.

I started using every opportunity I had to create positive energy. Think positive. Spread love, care. Be kind about each little thing, because small sands and drops of water create the persistent wave in a sea. I got rid of all my addictions. But I know the devil has a better degree than a PhD in making people do wrongs that create negative energy, so I never underestimate him anymore. He has lots of traps of desire or attachment to this world. Monotheism or understanding our communication with Allah or consciousness (as the book 'The Power of Now' talks about) are ways of creating detachment from this world. Evil is unconsciousness. Consciousness means living in the present and the present is light. You can use that light to do good things – that's positive energy. Unconsciousness is darkness.

Because of my spiritual beliefs now, I am not who I am labelled. I freed myself. I master patience, empathy. I create positive energy in my brain and heart. My brain chemicals are now balanced and I enjoy inner peace. Yes, there is still unconsciousness, but I try to be in the present to take unconsciousness away. How can you practice being conscious? As Muslims say, 'the remembrance of Allah' or if you want to say it in a different way I can say 'consciousness of creator'. Whatever you believe, be positive, because our mind and heart know what is consciousness. And He created all that exists, that we can see or cannot see, and all we know and all we don't know. You do not have to believe. Belief will come to you if you spread positive energy.

We are mentally ill, so what? We can still change this world – at least we can contribute something to the community, to the world. We also have positive energy. We can prove to this world that we are capable of something. I think one thing at a time, with patience with remembrance of 'the gift of now'. We are mentally ill, so what? We can seek good will as well. We can pursue knowledge. We can explore the whole world as well, and enjoy every present moment. Ask forgiveness from the creator. Forgive everyone. Forgive ourselves. Bloom as a flower. Be natural. We all have something special. We just have to try a little bit, as I am trying to explore that with you, while I am explaining it as well. The power of being together can create more positive energy. We can change this world.

We need a clear goal. Start with dreaming... or maybe something a bit 'realistic', but please dream. Hope is everything we have, so never lose that. Yeah, but how can we turn our dream into reality? Belief. Belief in our creator who is one. Belief that all power, success and wisdom comes according to His will. This is the essence of our true secret. We need to believe in ourselves and our abilities. Prophet Muhammad, peace and blessing be upon him, Allah says: "I am as my servant thinks I am, and I am with him if he calls for me...' (Bukhari and Muslim).

Then I think we just have to try to act on it. There is always a second chance when we try to do something good. Failure is the pillar of success. Learn from mistakes; not only your mistakes but also everyone's mistakes.

Learn to learn from mistakes – that's how we can overcome mistakes. We are already successful because we are all unique. We have already been given a chance to make mistakes like trillions of men from Adam till now. Constantly giving the idea to Adam (by Satan) that forbidden fruit is good brought us here in this world for many tests. To successfully go back to where we were, we just have to constantly generate positive ideas that create positive energy. Love to love is our idea. Love to be kind is our seed.

Growth
Roxy

I was a young child. I didn't speak out. I didn't understand it was wrong. I was too young. I was told not to speak out. I was only a child. I didn't know any better. I can never blame myself. It was never my fault. This was the worst thing that ever happened to me. I wish I could have changed it.

I was about sixteen years old when my parents divorced. I had a relationship breakdown with my boyfriend at the time. I attempted to take my own life. I thought it was the only way. It wasn't. I ended up in hospital. Guilt overwhelmed me as my family struggled to comprehend what I tried to do. I was then referred on to a clinical psychologist. I thought it was the worst thing that had happened to me.

When I was nineteen years old and in my second year of university I was hospitalized for severe eczema. My face was covered in blisters and half swollen. I was hospitalized because my Mum didn't know how to help me anymore. The doctors didn't know how to help either. They didn't know what it was. Old ladies who roamed the halls of the ward assumed I was a burns victim. I looked like Frankenstein. I truly believed I was a monster. My mental health suffered. I struggled with my university studies to the point where I thought I would have to drop out. I thought it was the worst thing that had happened to me.

I was twenty years old. As a third-year psychology student I was watching some lectures on psychological trauma. I also watched the Butterfly Effect. Something about this movie triggered memories of abuse. Ones I had suppressed. Ones I had tried to forget. My memories were so fragmented yet they were playing over and over, on repeat. I wanted them to stop but I couldn't make them disappear. It was in this moment I knew needed to see my psychologist. What if she thinks I'm crazy? What if she thinks I'm making this up? I've been seeing her for about four years and had never spoken about any of this.

I was struggling to speak out. I was starting to understand what happened. How wrong it was. How innocent I was. I was just doing what I was told to do. I didn't speak out at the time. I didn't. I tried to blame myself. I wanted to. But this was not my fault. This was the worst thing that ever happened to me. I wish I could have changed it. This was the worst thing that ever happened to me.

The initial processing of these memories was the hardest. I was seeing my psychologist almost weekly to receive ongoing support. My mental health had never been as low as it was at this time of my life. I was extremely depressed. Most days I thought about taking my own life. I was so sensitive and the little things people would do irritated me, even if they did these things unintentionally. Everything seemed too much. I had never gone through anything like this before. I didn't think that things were ever going to get better.

I was about twenty years old when I was hanging out with some of my old high school friends. One of them asked, "what's the worst thing that you have ever been through?". Everyone mentioned the death of our close high school friends. We all agreed. That was hard. I experienced that. But no one yet knew about what I had been through. It was then that I opened up and told them about my experiences of being abused as a child.

All of the blame. It was still there. I was struggling to speak out but starting to try. It was even harder than I thought it would be. Opening up to people, you know? After shutting my emotions off and suppressing everything for so many years. People were telling me how young I was and that I didn't know what I was doing. They told me it wasn't my fault and that they wished they would have known earlier. I tried my fucking hardest not to blame myself. I didn't want to anymore. But what happened to me is in no way my fault. This was the worst thing that happened to me and I wish I could've changed it.

I have recently graduated an Honours degree in Psychology with the career goal of becoming a clinical child psychologist. I am driven to help others through what I have been through. To help them understand that their trauma may be a part of their identity and it may impact them in ways often inexplicable at the time, but it does not need to define them. It's not an easy goal but I believe in myself whole heartedly. I know I can achieve this.

What I am most proud about is the fact that I am still here. My experiences have allowed me to become a more empathetic and understanding person, and they have driven me towards where I aim to be in life – helping other people. I'm proud that I made it through the darker times – not without struggles, but without those struggles I do not believe I would be the person I am today. Over time I've become more comfortable speaking to my close friends and family about my experiences. I know that there are people I can really trust who can offer the support that I need.

I was so young and naïve. It wasn't my fault. We all wished something happened earlier but it didn't. I can't blame myself. I don't need to anymore. This was not my fault. Even though it is hard I don't need to feel personally responsible. It was the worst thing that ever happened to me in my life so far.

But I am who am I because of what happened to me. My experiences have not broken me – they have built me. I do not wish I could have changed it.

Roxy is a Psychology Honours graduate who is aiming to be a child clinical psychologist. She enjoys seeing live music in her spare time, alongside reading, travelling and hanging out with her friends and family. Roxy is inspired by her own process of overcoming trauma and she aims to help others through similar experiences.

Trauma from a 'safe' space
Corey de Bruin

My family were dysfunctional and emotionally neglectful. As a result I've ended up playing the role of Hero. I've always helped and counselled friends, my brother and even my mother.

My parents fought continuously, and I had to protect my brother through all of it. I was also excluded at school, and in high school, I was bullied constantly. I left in year 11 and got a diploma in business and another in management. Then I started a computer science degree at university. I then dropped out.

When I began studying at university, I had some big problems, some of which I wasn't even aware of yet. The biggest one was not understanding at a fundamental level that to help others, you first need to help yourself. Another was the relationship I was about to get myself into, which fed off this lack of understanding. There were some hard consequences to this; burning out and dropping out of my course (there were other factors that contributed to this though) and the break-up of my first serious relationship (which I had grown dependent on, forming a co-dependent relationship).

When I began studying at university, I met and grew quite attached to one particular person who struggled with various mental health conditions along with some physical health and pain problems. Throughout that year I lost sight of any form of self-care and dedicated so much time to this complex relationship. I even ended up dropping out of my course and moving out of my share house at that time. I've always played the role of Hero so it would only make sense that I would now play that role again.

(Of course I didn't even think about it, it was instinctual.)

Over the entire period of this 'relationship' (around 1.5 years) I lost my sense of self. Most of that time is a blur, which isn't surprising because I came out of that relationship with a diagnosis of complex PTSD. (In all fairness I believe I had symptoms before that, but it wasn't enough for a 'clinical diagnosis'). I also had at least two admissions to hospital for attempted suicide during that time.

My time in the Psychiatric Emergency Care Centre/Unit (PECC), especially my second admission, was its own trauma, and I could have sworn I had died and gone to hell while I was there. As I've recounted countless times before, I was placed on TWO heavily sedating antipsychotics and a very potent Benzodiazepine, and still wasn't sleeping more than two hours per night. I was physically sick and couldn't eat, I couldn't sit still and had to either lay down or pace. Yet the nurses told me that I couldn't lie in bed, I couldn't lie down at all – yet the other patients were allowed to sleep during the day! (Apparently, the reason I couldn't sleep was that I was lying down during the day).

They told me that I HAD to eat even though I was just going to throw it back up anyway. (In my position, the way they said that was the same as forcing me to eat regardless of my wishes). One nurse was even rude enough to claim I was addicted and tolerant to 'Benzos' – this because I was prescribed the smallest dose of Xanax, despite the fact I rarely used it – and accused me of drug seeking.

Once I got out of that relationship and left the PECC, I spent three months laying on a sofa in my mother's garage because I could hardly go more than a few minutes without having panic attacks. I had to be drunk all the time and chain smoke just to be able to stop trembling, plus the alcohol seemed to help relax the rigidity in my muscles. At some point over those three months, my ex and her family came to collect my ex's belongings out of the garage where I was staying. Her father had words with me because my ex claimed I physically assaulted her (apparently I was drunk, and, that's why I couldn't remember it). This stuck with me, and I believed it for the better part of the following year – despite various therapists and friends who knew me and my ex quite well – stating that there was no way their story was true. It still occasionally haunts my mind and I believe it's even become a part of my complex PTSD.

Three months passed and I started my TAFE course sober. I told my GP I was getting off all drugs (and I managed to quit cold turkey with no withdrawals – not that this by any means should be seen as usual). Once I was clean, I remained that way for a few months.

I then went through a period where my thoughts were really bothersome and throughout the next year I experimented with Ketamine, MDMA, LSD, Weed, Xanax, and Oxynorm (high strength endone) in an attempt to quell the PTSD, the memories, and the depression. I stopped these after a few years of use with no problems. I miss them occasionally but, because I don't have the money to use and my mind is relatively stable, I choose not to continue to use.

Unfortunately, my ex decided to get back in contact. I decided, mistakenly, that maybe she had changed. I was wrong, luckily this time I had some perspective and I decided I wouldn't keep seeing her after just a few months, and I left in a reasonably good state.

Two years on and I received an ATAR equivalent score of 92. This despite spending my first exam period on three strong opioid medications and a nerve pain medication for wisdom tooth problems which were resolved over that Christmas period. (However, I'd spent months waiting to get any pain relief and then once I got it I spent close to a year waiting for the extraction. I can hardly remember the period when I was on those painkillers.)

I'm now advocating for suicide prevention and mental health programs. I've made it my life's work to 'help'. Isn't it funny how it's possible to take the roles that life provides and use them for good when they were initially harmful?

Looking back on these last few years, I learned that if you want to have healthy relationships and if you want to help others, you need to learn how to provide some distance and how to put yourself first. If you don't, others will need to pick up the pieces regularly, and you won't be any help to anyone.

I also learned that no matter how hard things seem, they can get better with the right help, but with the wrong support, they can get worse. And to remember, even when it seems pointless, once you get better you can advocate for those who are in the position you were in.

As somebody with a lived experience of suicidality and mental health conditions I want to ensure that others know that they aren't alone and that recovery is possible. Having experienced the difficulties with navigating the system, I want the world to be one where people speak out and the required help is available. Having finished my HSC equivalency with an ATAR of 92, I plan to attend university from 2020 to study a social work degree.

Journey Out of Madness
Jennie Somerville

You've got to push for recovery, it doesn't just happen.

I am a 'survivor of psychiatry' (2006) and more recently, an early breast cancer survivor (2018).

The difference between my two survivor stories is that, with mental ill-health I survived the treatments and mental health system of care (psychiatry), and with early breast cancer I survived the disease. It should not be that way – interventions that actually end up more damaging to the patient than the illness itself.

So, what happened to me?

At 48, I was working full time, studying Sociology part time, raising my teenage daughter and renovating a home with my partner, a clinical psychologist. Life was good. About that time, I began experiencing severe symptoms of an (undiagnosed) early menopause. Insomnia, agitation, panic and fear. Soon I was unable to cope with the normal demands of life and could not work or concentrate on study. To my despair, my daughter returned to live with her father, as I was unable to parent her. A terrible situation for a teenage girl; she was forming her own identity, while I was rapidly losing mine.

A psychiatrist diagnosed major depression and prescribed a cocktail of drugs and Electroconvulsive Therapy (ECT). My family were at their wits end as my personality changes were completely out of character, and there was no history of mental problems in our family. My relationship floundered under the strain and ultimately ended. I became paranoid and experienced strange beliefs (for example, that I was an illegal immigrant). One night, I fled the house in my pyjamas. Finally, after six months, I found myself living with the diagnosis of late-onset schizophrenia (later to be proved incorrect). This diagnosis had profound and catastrophic consequences for my family and me. Life as I knew it ended and I moved into unchartered and undesired territory: that of female psychiatric patient.

My elderly parents courageously took me in, as I had nowhere to live. But this was destined to fail. My mother's health was poor and she was already a carer for my father, who was in the early stages of dementia. Ultimately, after a year or so, the stress of managing my condition – and the implications of living with them – became untenable. My siblings called a halt to it, and I was placed in the care of the mental health system. I spent about four years (in total) living in a series of dysfunctional and unsafe group homes, and in transitional living accommodation, sharing mostly with males.

I had frequent hospitalisations, some spent in solitary confinement. Once, in the community, I experienced a toxic side effect of medications through mismanagement, and almost died, ending up in the intensive care unit. I was sexually assaulted by another patient during one of my admissions to a sub- acute/low supervision unit, and some years later when I had left the mental health system, I lodged a Victims of Crime application and was successful in receiving a small pay-out. It was validation for me for the abuse and negligence I had suffered as a public psychiatric patient. Today, I advocate for single sex wards.

There was no therapy or psychosocial rehabilitation of any form during this time. Worse, I had no advocate, family or otherwise, in a system where I was totally cast adrift. I resoundingly 'fell through the cracks'. By now my daughter (to her credit and sheer tenacity) had successfully completed university and was living overseas. I rarely saw her anyway, and after diagnosis and the ensuing separation, lost the bond we had. I guess the stigma and the shame of having a severely mentally ill mother was difficult to integrate. She finally sought help herself, through ARAFMI (now Mental Health Carers NSW) and then private therapy. No help, education or support was ever offered to her, or to us as a family, by the mental health system.

Finally, I ended up in an aged care facility. I was 53. I was told I would need care for the rest of my life and would never work again or live in the community. All hope seemed lost, but little did I realise my life was about to change in radical and transformative ways.

To my delight, I had my own private room with ensuite and had no chores or cleaning up after other residents to do, as had been the case in mental health care. I was living with mainly frail older women, not men. I felt safe and the staff were kind. Our meals were provided. But best of all, I met a highly skilled and compassionate music psychotherapist, Kirstin, on the staff, who somehow gained my trust and offered me therapy. I was scared and sceptical and very shut down, but what did I have to lose? No one had ever taken an interest in me clinically, so I didn't believe I deserved or would benefit from help. I felt so worthless and disabled by my illness. Nonetheless, Kirstin had thrown me a life line, and I tentatively took hold of it.

Well in sum, after three years of music psychotherapy and the stable stress-free living situation, I was able to leave the aged hostel facility to set up my own flat in a small mountain village west of Sydney. By mutual consent, I severed ties with the mental health team when my psychiatrist agreed to take me off the last of my medications. I returned to study the next year, in 2007, and gained a Mental Health Cert IV (with distinction).

Today, I live a meaningful and happy life in a regional town. I have been fortunate to have received some small inheritances along the way, which has greatly enhanced my recovery journey. I had a brief relapse in 2017 (which took me completely by surprise!) but I stabilised and recovered quickly after hospitalisation and medication, which I'm slowly coming off with the support of my general practitioner. I realised I needed more help, and now have a Flourish Australia worker, whose support I value. I still see a psychotherapist (not Kirstin), as ongoing therapy and the benefits it brings in terms of insight and clarification has been at the core of rebuilding my life. I work hard at maintaining my physical and mental health (adequate sleep, gym, dancing, good nutrition and spending time with friends). I try to take every opportunity that comes my way and I never, ever take life for granted.

Last year I completed the Intentional Peer Support (IPS) Core Training and plan to become a teacher of lived experience and recovery in universities and TAFE, after I complete a Certificate IV in Training and Assessment. I hope what happened to me as a patient – damaged not healed by mental health interventions – will never happen to anyone else. This is one reason I speak openly about my experience.

My daughter is 41 now, married and living in Ireland; she gained her PhD and works as an academic there. Oh yes, and I have a beautiful six-year-old grandson who I Skype!

Somehow, we all got across the line, after such devastating losses, and life is good.

Jennie Somerville trained as a teacher in the late 60s, married and emigrated to Canada in 1970. Discovering that teaching children was not for her, she studied counselling and worked as a Family Court Counsellor in The Provincial Court of British Columbia. On return to Australia in 1980 Jennie worked for NSW Health as a social welfare worker in regional hospitals. Today Jennie is self-employed, working as an Intentional Peer Support Practitioner and Mental Health Peer Educator and Consultant.

Have you ever seen a bull doing backstroke?
E. S. Katz

CW: drugs, death, some discussions of suicide

While writing this I am acutely aware of the multi-faceted and often chronic issues people, and some of my very close friends, face every single day. It's hard not to reflect and even chastise myself with the traditional 'imposter syndrome' caveats: "They have the REAL problems, you have no place writing about this", "you have so much going for you YOU can't be [insert condition here]", or even "you've gotten past this now, your issues are over – go and get on with things".

Considering all that, my motivations for writing this piece are threefold: a) I have recently suffered through a completely destabilizing FEP event (First Episode Psychosis) caused by the use of illicit drugs; b) this event prompted a deeper reflection and 'existential' complication on my overall mental health and approach to life, and finally; c) I find writing cathartic.

My reasons for taking the drugs were varied. I had gone to live overseas (for reasons I will come to shortly) and had visited Amsterdam, as probably a lot of young 20-somethings do, and had tried psychedelics: specifically psilocybin mushrooms.

For one reason or another I hoped to undergo some sort of profound experience: you can read the multitude of content online about 'trips', enlightenment etc, but there are great difficulties in discussing this topic, with regards to legality, the subjectivity involved with unfiltered 'recounts' from anonymous people on the internet, and general misinformation and fear-mongering. I ended up going through psychosis which SANE

Australia defines as a mental disorder where a person loses the capacity to tell what's real from what isn't.

Describing psychosis as a sensory experience is difficult, particularly in a short span of writing. To put it simply, for me it was like being in a video-game or virtual reality of sorts. I was still 'me' to some extent, though the ridiculous or absurd becomes physically real. The experience was completely staggered, both immediately after I took the drugs, then for about two weeks – and then around two months afterwards as I cycled through medical or psychiatric wards, journeyed back home an erratic and delusional wreck, and found some antipsychotic prescription that didn't leave me drooling and incoherent. If this all sounds confronting I apologise (as I did profusely and often to all my friends and family that had come to help me in the aftermath).

I think the best way to describe myself, to the general public, is that I am not some pseudo-intellectual mystic or new-age shaman and I did not expect to reach nirvana, neither am I a habitual drug user, though I was smoking, drinking and using marijuana more regularly than at any other point in my life.

I had a safe living environment growing up, and what I would consider a good loving family; though as with all families there were dysfunctions, angst and expectations, and a growing need for negotiating boundaries and feeling respected. I think you can be for all intents and purposes safe, in a first-world nation, and still not feel 100%, though I acknowledge my privileged status.

Additionally, I thought of potential side-effects and risks: I took some of the general precautions beforehand (being around friends in a physically safe environment etc and so on) though there are always more risks. At this point some people might just flippantly respond with "drugs are bad", or "that's illegal, so you deserve whatever happens", or even just "you're an idiot", but this is a mired topic at best. To answer the questions along the lines of "you had no clue what you were doing, what if you died?", my only answer was that to some extent, I didn't really care. Ambivalence is one of my favourite words, and on the topic of life and death it definitely suits. I had been born, and it was that inertia that kept me going, rather than 'pulling' force. Newton's first law as often stated: an object at rest stays at rest and an object in motion stays in motion with the same speed and in the same direction, and I looked at drugs as nothing more than a small catalyst. Additionally... this was not heroin, or some dark addictive 'cut' substance that is nothing more than a 'life-ruiner'. I think classifying drugs is important; there are levels.

This might sound immature to some, melodramatic to others, but it felt, and in some ways still feels today, like the general pathos of my approach to life. I don't think I'd ever have actively killed myself, and wouldn't say I thought about suicide any more than the usual idle thoughts people have – what if I walk to close to that ledge, imagine that bus hit me while I'm crossing the street – but I just felt a bit blasé about going on with life as we know it.

Before this, my childhood, teens, early 20s, I felt like I'd always been a bull in a china shop.

When I hit issues, insecurities or 'cringe-moments', in my past I dealt with it by just lowering my head and smashing-it-out, OR charging so hard into other things to stay distracted from bigger 'existential' problems. Everything was a fight, and everyone a potential enemy. I knew if I stopped for any given time, I would just overthink myself into submission.

"Come on", "She'll be right", "Let's smash out the next task", was my mantra.

Perseverance was what I perceived to be my super-power. I wasn't overly smart, or strong, tough etc, but I just kept going, I was stubborn, persistent, or as my family would say, a 'doer'. Sure I'd feel sad, or more often than not angry, and in the quiet moments I would be assailed by the weight of the stupid things I'd said or done, but I was always busy with some task or another: university, work, chores and helping family or constant social engagements. Constant noise deafened the 'blah', but slowly the punch-drunkenness set in and things generally just got muggy.

I ran away to a far-off new place for a variety of reasons, but for the most part it was to combat this mugginess: a feeling of isolation, of emotional fatigue, of feeling unwanted and unloved, as well as an overwhelming need to just shut people up around me, make a fresh start. As probably a lot of people, much younger than me go through as well, I was also eager to just split away and prove what I could do… even to myself. I was safely wading in the shallows. I had an idea of what I was capable of, though also some bluff and sincere ignorance.

In short, I made a go of things and it worked for a little while, I tackled some challenges with vim and vigour, and handled others about as well as that same young bull turning to synchronized swimming. I was drowning. The drug trip was probably an ill-timed bucket list event, but also a first step in trying to find, or create, a better way of being *myself.*

In some ways it did. I don't think 'mental breakdown' is a real diagnosed condition, but colloquially I think this sums up my distressing experience at this point, and it really showed me that it was time for things to change.

The phrases 'mental health issue', or M.H. distress seemed a bit ubiquitous when they first hit my ears as I always thought everyone goes through issues in the day-to-day: I believe everyone can feel sad, or needy or anxious, but the general ethos is to 'soldier on' or 'sort it out', and then move on to happiness and fulfillment. My not so original opinion is that the topic of mental health is a little like education, or parenting: it's something that everyone has an experience with (whether positive or negative) and therefore everyone feels justified in having a 'stance' on its application, quality and resolution.

I'm reminded of another meme, of an imaginary conversation a young man has with someone from his life, probably a family member, which goes something like:

"You're just depressed because you stay in your bedroom all day instead of travelling the world".

[Young Man takes selfie in front of a Sphynx] "Cool now I'm depressed in Egypt".[1]

It's taken quite a while, around two years on various antipsychotics, weight gain, really low-points, self-doubt, and directionless anger and shame, as well as a lot of 'work' to finally feel 'normal'. I have been seeing a 'psych' (mental health worker) regularly to continue negotiating this recovery process. I still have bouts of dissociation – a sense that things

---

1 *Depressed in Egypt [meme]. 2018. Retrieved from www.reddit.com/r/FunnyandSad/comments/82133k/well_lad/*

around me are not real, or sometimes feeling 'outside' of my body – and I think these are really important things for people to learn a bit more about. I was super worried for a long time about those 'ego-death' symptoms the gurus of the web come up with, but I've come to learn these are actually really natural and safe states. I still feel isolated in many ways. At the current time I don't feel like I have a confidante I can share openly with, but I do have some friends and good people around me.

I still have a long way to go for self-growth, but I've had some small successes in the various spheres of my life: building up to working full-time again, renegotiating friendships and 'toxic' relationships, as well as changing those habitual behaviours within myself that just aren't conducive to a peaceful existence (for myself or others). I tend towards the negative, so I try to temper my bias with the words of my pysch – he tells me to reflect on my habits or past actions and make changes if I need to, but to always do these things with kindness. Try to avoid pressure words like "I should be doing that…", "I must change…" and try to be a bit more flexible. I always loved Bruce Lee, so maybe its poignant to include "become *like* water my friend", rather than just *IN* the water.

I think the most valuable insight my story has taught me is to not leave things until you're drowning. Don't just think you seek help when you're at your lowest point; everyone is entitled to help even if they're just feeling down one day. If things aren't feeling right, I tell myself sometimes it's okay to just slow down, take my time and be a bit delicate with the fine china. And my head.

A 20-something Greek-Australian first generation immigrant, proud social justice warrior, casual writer, hopeful nihilist, polyam, aspiring Saint-Walker and superhero enthusiast. Trying to make the world better one iterant unrestrained economically-left meme or obscure quote at a time.

"Justice and power must be brought together, so that whatever is just may be powerful, and whatever is powerful may be just" ~Blaise Pascal

"VOICES"
Margaret Lincoln

My hope now lies in quietude. It's true. My brain and soul have been ill-affected by more stress than a bodily organ can take, and still maintain its parts in an orderly fashion. I'm told I haven't lost my God-given intelligence and my (also God-given) intuition is stronger than ever if I listen to the whisperings. I've learnt so much through years of physical illness, disability, disordered emotional and cognitive systems and, yes, even the experiences of literally dying and surviving.

Voices tell me I should be otherwise than I am. The haranguing, cruel hallucinatory voices of others now long gone: the horrific images; the voices of society telling us what we 'should' be like now at our age; the voices even of loved ones who refuse to hear the truth of my experience, and the voices of doctors and nurses who do not understand the ways of a brain-and-heart too hurt. Even the 'recovery movement' of other people who've lived with mental distress tells me that I should be leading others into their own recovery. I'm done with grasping desperately to continue to work, order life and environment, maintain equilibrium, perform basic function. I'll be beside. I'll sit with some in their torment. I'll help meet the needs denied in hospitals. I'll take the hands of others to a long moment of respite, but I'll not lead and strive now.

My sad father had a severely disordered mind. He told me I was like him and needed quiet environments in which to live and work. I so desperately didn't want to be like my father that I drove myself for fifty years. I've been to worldly heights and mixed with so-called powerful people. The work has at times been glamorous – ultimately empty, but glamorous. The body and mind can take no more driving and striving, achieving and leading. Some of my own dishevelment comes from not heeding the paternal voice spoken so many years gone. Yes, I am like my father in that my nerves are worn and shredded. My body is considerably broken. I need now to acknowledge and live the wisdom in his advice.

In all this cacophony of 'should' and tyranny, my very own voice tells me that my hope lies in quiet living – the authentic voice tells me this. I can listen to God talking to me in His loving way, guiding me, teaching me. In that I can find my recovery, peace and rightly-ordered mind and actions. I can no longer let all the voices of 'other' goad and drive me, determining my life.

Today, my brain actually connected with my feelings to make the idea whole. I can think through each moment in quietude. Now, God helps me act to build a life, in its final third, of steadiness and gentle living of lessons hard learned. The clement strength of my own voice tells me this is my style of recovery. It's how to come back to myself from continual high distress and living voices foreign to me. May you, my friends, my fellows, find your authentic voice to guide you to your place of wholeness.

Margaret lives with a range of physical and mental health conditions. In her retirement, she is passionate about being an advocate beside people living with mental health issues. Margaret thoroughly enjoys voluntary reading with primary school children. Classical music is one of her sustaining activities. She also likes conversations with precious friends, water exercise and 'doona' days.

From B to AA
Samantha

I have heard it said that hindsight is an exact science. My story could be evidence that our system is more broken than any individual's mental health. One could argue we are products of an iatrogenic system. This story has been a search to find the answers to three essential questions: who am I? where do I belong? and what am I meant to do? For me, life has been a process of finding true meaning. A journey to discovering happiness is just an external facade used by people who know no different. It is through Inner Joy, Peace and Love that true meaning has come. Not without trial. This story is a story of pain, a story of acceptance and a story of hope. A story of spiritual awakening from the outside in, then later, the inside out.

Samantha lay her baby girl in the cot after having fed her. She watched and wept, feeling a complete disconnect from the joy she had anticipated this baby would bring. "This is not how it's meant to be." All her life she felt things that didn't align with her expectations. Expectations imposed on her by her family, friends, society and then internalised and lived from. She was meant to be happy. She had been fighting to pull happiness in from the outside. The first time she smoked pot, at 14, she felt it, a sense of relief from the pressures on her to perform in a world full of actors. She felt it when she received love and acceptance from men, boys. She expected to feel it from this new life she had given birth to. Her desperation had led her here, a mental health ward for mothers and their babies. Darkness overwhelmed her. Hopeless. In this state of desperation she fell to her knees, questioning the idea of God. Her nana had gone to church at one point but she tried to end her life. "If there is anyone there, I need help." A knock on her door alarmed her but the medication had numbed her senses to what this meant. A woman from the hospital's chapel appeared with a blanket, not understanding the implications of this prayer, nor realising it was even a prayer, this visit and gift of a blanket was an immediate answer to a prayer she didn't even know she was praying. The blanket was inscribed 'wish upon a star'...

As a teenager Samantha discovered the best way to run from the alien in her mind (ego) was intoxication. Her need to get approval from the authorities in her life meant a double life, the facade failing when she could no longer abide by mother's rules and branched out on her own. Seventeen and living free! Freedom soon became imprisonment as her mind needed protection from the realities she found herself in. She inhabited a home with a man who dealt hard drugs and had implanted a camera in the shower, connecting it to a monitor in his bedroom. Her mind could not cope with this reality, drugs or no drugs, psychosis was imminent.

Within a year she had three hospitalisations for drug induced psychosis, which resulted in the Bipolar label. Mania and a disconnect with reality called for a needle in the bum. Reality was protected by the cloud of medication which she was told and believed, for a time, to be the solution. Deep within she knew she was searching for love and connection, for belonging. Many nights manically scribing these intuitive revelations showed her there was a part of this world that was unseen, and seemingly ignored by most of the others acting in the show of life. But she seemed to have no option, the pain on her mother's face resulting from her erratic behaviours didn't lie. She subscribed to the diagnosis and dove into the solution the medical fraternity presented to her. Classes in CBT (Cognitive Behavioural Therapy), emotional regulation, mindfulness as well as taking the prescribed medication. She continued, for years, to balance her internal state with prescribed medication, pot and alcohol. Imprisoned in her own mind, and now chained to a system supposedly designed to help one's mind get fixed. Think your way into a sound mind! Simple.

Still searching for love, Samantha, with her now one-year-old, found herself dating a man whose parents went to church. The unconditional love of this family highlighted something she was missing. One Sunday morning she woke up with an urgency to go to church. They jumped at the chance to bring this desolate young mother to a service. That same love and acceptance was received from this church family. Believing in Jesus was a no brainer (which was good as her mind was clearly broken). She knew she needed Divine help and the promise of the Holy Spirit to guide her was too great an offer to pass by. This confession, unbeknownst to her was her first spiritual rebirthing experience.

She was prompted by the loving compassion of the pastors, not only to give up the pot but also to attend Bible College. The hunger she felt for more of this Unconditional Love was growing. She gave up the pot and worked her way toward getting off medication. This new family was where she belonged. Samantha was not known to do things in half measures. The following years saw her pursue a degree in teaching, running a children's outreach ministry and travelling overseas on multiple mission trips. Her ingrained need for external approval was still running her life. She burnt out. The pressure, imposed by herself and her perception of what was expected of her as a Christian, was too much. She needed a change.

Finding a similar church to one that she was reborn in, she appeared to be taking time to heal. She was teaching in a pre-kindy, parenting her now teenage daughter, studying psychology, seeing a Christian Counsellor, a psychologist and a life coach. Her drinking was progressively increasing but it wasn't working anymore to calm her mind and her emotions. She questioned this God she had learned to love. Did He really die on a cross for me to feel this crap? She wanted out. She was done but suicide was selfish and she was a mum. But she needed something, pot smoking returned. Having done enough psychotherapy she recognised the addictive behaviour. Four days straight, she could see she was going backwards. A friend suggested a 12 step fellowship.

In these rooms she heard her story. She saw that the Power of God worked in people's lives, regardless of the name they used for that Power. She began to have her mind opened. The love and compassion was authentic due to the vulnerability necessary to recover. Success was built in these peoples' lives from a place of utter desperation, which is where she was at. These AAs had an answer. The religious pride and people pleasing wouldn't fly with these guys, they knew the tricks. These games she had played her whole life, they knew all too well. She could be real with these people, her people. The deception and delusion that Samantha had played her whole life was merely a façade. She worked hard at this recovery journey, with the desperation of a dying woman. Through this program for living she saw the causes and conditions that lead her to her knees in a drunken state in her living room could be overcome. This prayer, as sincere as the one in the mental health ward, was the beginning of her God revealing to her an authentic way to live her life. This time, from the inside out.

This story hopes to highlight the humanity of living with an insane mind. I hope it highlights the broken system we live in that can only be healed and made whole by the individuals within it becoming whole, from the inside out. A spiritual way of life is not weakness – we need an inner connectedness with Power to truly be able to connect with ourselves and the people about us. Life is not easy! The reality of my internal life, my thinking, feeling and spiritual self and how I interact with people and in systems can be a daily struggle. But I am doing it. I am now experiencing periods of contentment and peace amidst the chaos of life that I never thought possible. Not because of, nor in spite of, the problems in the world, but because of the people within it. The people who, along my journey have showed me true love and compassion. Those who have loved me when I couldn't love myself. Those who loved me enough to call me on my crap and show me that even with that ugly side they could love me. Those who, when I was unable to, could help me see what I needed to see. Even in the uncomfortable times. Life is messy. Life is beautiful. It cannot be either or, it is always both.

On a journey to discovering who I am, where I belong and what I am meant to do. I have recently launched into a business venture to educate and teach from a lived experience perspective. Advocating for the rights of the individual at a systemic level with the individual being at the centre. I enjoy reading and writing and hanging out with my tribe. Loving living life one day at a time and enjoy being around water.

For Sanity's Sake
TigerSpirit

In a way, I could relate to Robin Williams. He kept his depression hidden, only letting people see the humorous side of him. I do that with so many things. Very rarely do I vent on social media about what my concerns are. People don't need to know my sob story. My mother taught me something a very long time ago, "Laugh and the world laughs with you, cry and you cry alone". She also taught me to try to see the positive side of everything; and although I struggled with this at times, my humour, through various experiences, became warped enough that I COULD see the positive side of the most tragic circumstances, although I've learned, for the sake of sensitivity to others, to best keep darker humour to myself.

But I'm not here to write about this. I want to share how my personality as a whole developed into one that struggles to act normal at times: if truth be told, I'm not normal, far from it. With all that I've had to deal with in my life, it's just impossible to be normal, and if there is one thing I've learned in recent years – everything… every little experience, positive or negative, changes a person, sometimes in a good way, sometimes not.

I was a big baby at birth. According to my mother thirteen pounds, eight ounces is a very big baby (although over the years, I've heard tell of bigger babies from friends). My mother never let me live that down, OR the fact that I tore her open… I can't deny or confirm if it was caused by me though, even if my mum was still alive. Mum would often joke that after I was born, she demanded that she have a coffee and a cigarette before they do anything else, so they complied and mum got her coffee and cigarette, and after she had a sip of her coffee and a puff of her smoke, the doctor asked her, "now, are you ready for the stitches?"

"WHAT STITCHES?!?" Apparently I tore her to her belly button: she had a scar from her vagina to her belly button, and she'd show it to me often. She never regretted having me, and she wore that scar proudly – always showing it off to whomever wanted to hear the story.

She never let me live down the fact that I was an 'April Fool' baby. On the first of April, at around 1am, mum seemingly went into labour. The doctor was dragged out of bed to come help deliver me. Apparently though, I was in the wrong position and not ready to come out. The doctor manually turned me around, and I turned back, he attempted to turn me again, and again I turned back to my original position. After a couple hours of this, he grumpily said to my mum, "SHE'S NOT READY! Go home and don't come back till she's ready to come out!"

It was another five days before I decided to come out. With mum often reminiscing about these two stories, I think that helped develop my wicked sense of humour, and the antics of April Fool's day became a tradition in our home. These were the good times, times that helped me learn to stay positive about the dark times that intermingled.

I was born with a twisted bowel and mum had been warned by the doctor that delivered me that IF I live past the first two years of my life, I would need an operation as my bowels were badly twisted, and most children around that time, in the 1960s, didn't live very long with this.

Mum struggled with me in those early months. For starters, I was allergic to her breast milk. I was also allergic to any formula they tried me on, nothing would stay down. After every idea they had failed, one nurse who had lived in the country, suggested they try goat's milk. This worked. I believe it was the only thing that kept me alive during those early months. Mum told me I cried a lot during that time as I was constantly in pain, but there was nothing she, or the doctors, could do.

When it came time for solids, the next big issue was finding food that I could digest. I threw up after every meal, nothing would stay down. It didn't help that mum did eventually seek out paediatrics in regards to the surgery that I needed but they didn't believe her. The tests they did (mostly barium enemas which can be highly traumatising for a young child) didn't (or couldn't) show the twist in the bowel and through trial and error, mum finally worked out the foods I could eat; bland steamed vegetables, white meat, and of course the goats milk.

Around the time I was almost ready for school, a miracle happened. My twisted bowels SOMEHOW sorted itself out, but the diagnosis now became a severe blockage in the bowel. The doctors couldn't be sure where, and because they didn't want to admit defeat, they decided unanimously they would just tell my mother that I was psychosomatic and should see a psychiatrist.

At around six years of age, mum took me to one. I learned that he wouldn't be poking and prodding me like others, so I was able to relax a bit and played a game of chess with myself (a common habit with me around this age as I had no friends, a side effect of spending most of my youth in hospitals). Whilst I did this, the psychiatrist would ask me questions. I remember the chess game, but don't remember the conversation. Mum later told me that after roughly an hour, the psychiatrist escorted me out of the office and said to my mum, "Here take her! Mentally, she's perfect and very intelligent, whatever issues she has are definitely physical!"

Apparently, whilst playing my game of chess, I asked the psychiatrist, "Is this what you do as a job? Sit around all day charging people to ask them really stupid questions." Another moment that my mother amusingly never let me live down.

By the age of twelve, I'd had enough. The doctors wanted to do another barium enema to see what was happening, but I went into hysterics, so they cancelled the test. By this time, I was getting suppositories after every meal, enemas once a week, and barium enemas routinely every month. I understood medical terminology that I shouldn't have known at the same age that other children were just learning to read. Doctors and examinations meant poking and prodding in the most painful ways.

It's no wonder that to this day, over four decades on, I still find hospitals traumatising to the point that I have panic attacks every time I go into one, and my regular GP is lucky if she sees me three times a year. At age 12, I pleaded with my mum to never take me to another doctor again. She agreed. The treatments all stopped, but the physical pain continued.

Roughly a year later, I was able to make my very first controlled bowel motion. I was so excited about it, I left school after my visit to the toilet that day to tell my mum: for me, a bowel motion WAS a big deal.

Over the years, I've learned EVERY home remedy there is to learn to heal whatever part of the anatomy needs treating. I often won't see the doctor until I've recovered – I only go in to let them know that I'd recently been sick, and tell them how I've treated it. I think my doctor likes it when I see her, my visits are almost always short and sweet.

That past trauma affects me in other aspects of my life. I don't handle confrontation well. I have been bullied by various departments over the years which has caused me a great deal of anxiety, which in turn affects me physically. Every time I feel stress, my blood pressure rises and triggers chest pains.

My negative experiences also aggravate my depression. I refuse to seek help for my mental health, as past experiences have taught me that doctors are more trouble than they're worth. I hide my pain, my anxiety, my depression and all that my trauma has caused. I show the world my sense of humour instead. I deal with my stress through prayers, writing, reading, colouring, crafts; my fur babies, and more recently, listening to podcasts.

These activities might not work on others or cure my mental issues, but they keep me calm and sane.

TigerSpirit is a poet and short story writer who plans to write some books in the future. Most of her writings are inspired by her past; even those that are mostly fiction have some basis of her own personal experiences. She doesn't put blame on past events or family, but instead has embraced it and knows that she's the person she is today because of all that has happened to her. View her work here: tigerspirits.wordpress.com.

About Hope
Michael Hill

Introduction

This is a story from my experiences about hope that I presented to our inaugural Mental Health Peer Work Cert IV class at Nowra. It was our first assessment. I had written another story before this that was basically my disaster story. I had told my disaster story many times in gory detail at support group meetings, but it was brought to my attention that as a peer worker my job is to convey something more useful, something that has been learned on the way. So here is the 'take two' story. (For the full experience, you may wish to download and listen to the song that was played at the conclusion: "Where My Heart Will Take Me" by Russell Watson.)

Almost 10 years ago I had a number of very traumatic life-changing experiences with my mental and physical health. At that time, I thought I was going to lose everything that was important to me, my job, my marriage, my home and much more.

Fortunately, over the years and with help from both my support group and my GP I have managed to:

-       keep my job and, after struggling at first, I regained the respect of my colleagues, which actually took quite a few years to do;

-       build a better relationship with my wife, who I am back with now and asks my advice on lots of things including mental health (not that I am always right! lol.);

- reassess and redirect my life to make it more meaningful. With regard to this I have left what would be classed as a good Council job on my own terms to allow me to work in mental health peer support. I enrolled in the Mental Health Peer Work Cert IV which I am sure will help me to use what I have gone through in order to help others. This is something I am much more interested in and is much more satisfying;

- gain paid employment with a great peer focused organisation called Flourish where I am able to learn and further use my experiences with mental health to support others in their recovery.

In the past nine years I have given my story quite a few times as an important healing tool for myself and others at support meetings. Now I have been challenged by doing this course to tell my story a totally different way. So, while I have told my story before, this is the first time I have given this version:

I am not going to go through the horrible and lengthy story of my mental and physical free fall in any detail. Instead I wanted to focus on a message about using hope and developing a positive habit of thinking and talking in a specific way day to day which I have found by experience to be a very helpful tool.

The trick

An example: I might maintain a hope to be treated the same as everyone else in my daily work life without the stigma associated with having depression or panic attacks.

In reality I have found this just may not happen… but things will never change or get better if I am continually thinking "I am *never* going to be treated as normal because they all know about my embarrassing past".

A habit of thinking this way will pretty well guarantee it won't happen any time soon.

People do notice even when it is not spoken. In particular I have found that rather than try to think positive thoughts all the time, which really is impossible, it is much easier to stop yourself when a bad thought arises. At first nothing changes but in developing this habit the space will eventually be automatically filled with something better. People around you will notice and appreciate your hopeful presence.

HOPE is a tool that is universal.

I don't even have to have had depression or panic attacks to use it – anyone can. Without trying or realising it, many people use hope every day in their lives.

So, for a theoretical example imagine you are the pilot of a jumbo jet (and by the way my favourite TV show is Air Crash Investigations!!)

As a good jet pilot, you might take off and without even thinking too much go through your checks etc. while having a hopeful attitude that your destination will be reached on time without major problems.

For a pilot it is a habit that is generally positive without much conscious thought about it. But if for no reason your thought train went along the lines of…

Geez I wonder… did that mechanic fill the fuel tanks properly? Maybe the gauge is wrong? He looked a bit sus. Maybe he tampered with the gauge and for no particular reason he's out to get me! They are all out to get me!! Hmmm…

It would probably affect your thinking big time and therefore your ability as a pilot to fly!!

So, these examples give a hint of how people will treat us if we have a habit of hooking into negative thoughts or saying negative things that may not even be true. My last example is another real-life story of someone who has a great way of using hopeful thinking.

A friend's story

This is a friend I met who many years ago who lived at a group home. He has allowed me to convey a part of his story. He is always extremely positive in spite of a number of serious health challenges. He was determined and had a hopeful goal of living in his own place. Many of his friends including myself tried to talk him out of this believing it was unrealistic. We were wrong. He has now had his own place for a number of years.

Next, he wanted to get a car and again many of his friends thought this to be unattainable, even reckless. This time I knew he was determined and as a learner someone would always be in the car as well. It took a while but he got his licence with no mishaps. He has now got a car to go with his licence and has not put a dent in it after driving for years.

His attitude made the difference and got him there in spite of his health challenges and much opposition.

So, to conclude

I believe it is very important that we all continue to develop the habit of monitoring what we think and say, spotting the bad stuff and in doing so, eventually managing to keep a hopeful attitude without even trying. One nice side effect is that people tend to hang around more if your conversation is reasonably hopeful. That is not to say that everything is rosy and perfect, shit still happens! But this is a tool to help get our thoughts going in a direction that is useful.

I hope that now, as a peer worker, the habit of spotting and discrediting unhelpful thoughts and talk (that sometimes may not even be true) will make space for more hopeful and helpful options.

I would like to finish by reminding you to listen to the song mentioned at the start. When I listen to this song it is very hard not to feel a bit more positive. I hope you find this also.

And thanks for reading my story.

Michael was until recently employed by Shoalhaven Council building various IT networks including radio, data, and security for projects such as the Illawarra Emergency Management Centre. Michael had planned a trip around Australia until finding the Cert IV in Mental Health Peer Work and was soon employed by Flourish Australia as a Peer Worker. Michael is very excited to be part of what he sees will be a revolution in Mental Health work, i.e. Peer Work.

My Story Is Not Over Yet
Sharon Lomnicki

My eyes are still shut, I feel the light coming through the groggy veil. Fuck, it's morning. Fuck, how am I going to do this, how am I going to get through the day? I turn over, squeeze my eyes shut and wish to drift back off so I don't have to face the accusing thoughts, the smothering guilt, the constant pain in my heart pounding out of my chest. Every single negative event I could possibly conjure up that I have experienced in my life comes banging and hammering to the forefront of my mind, reliving all the humiliation, the pain, the isolation, the rejection, the betrayal, the lies, the taunts, the harassment, the physical and emotional abuse that has been inflicted upon me. I steel myself for the fight, I just have to make it through the day, minute by minute, hour by hour, until the safety of night wraps me in its darkness and a slight reprieve befalls me. Broken sleep, insomnia comes to stay, at least it is night and I can be alone. It is too hard to burden another human being with my melancholia.

You see when I'm 'normal', when I'm 'me', I'm at peace with it all. I've done a lot of work on myself: mindfulness, numerous visits to psychologists, doctors, psychiatrists, counsellors, meditation, aromatherapy, supplements, etc… etc… I'm quite optimistic by nature, fun loving and friendly, but all that goes by the wayside when the dark cloud of depression slowly creeps its cold prickly arms around me; a day or two (which is the norm now) I can handle, but a few years ago I was convinced by a well-meaning friend that I didn't need meds, I was doing ok and just needed to eat healthily and take St John's Wort. I told no one and gave it a go…

I diligently tapered back my medication, an SSRI at the time. I had the normal ups and downs of everyday life and coped quite well. I had a loving husband and two beautiful children, a roof over our heads and food on the table. I had been told that the correct way to wean off meds was to do it slowly: a few months of half a tablet, then a quarter tablet, then an eighth of a tablet, replaced with St John's Wort, a natural herb reputed for aiding clinical depression. I should have known, I had tried to go off my meds before over the years.

Clinical Depression. As I write this, I am in my 50th year, I was 24 when I first saw a psychiatrist. My life was spiralling out of control, drugs and alcohol were the self-medications that numbed the pain and deep self-loathing I felt. Every judgement that was thrown at me ate away at my soul. I broke up with my partner of eight years and lost the house we purchased. I worked in a coffee shop, the boss was not a kind man and the staff took delight in bullying me and taking advantage of me whenever they could. I would go to work, and everything was a blur. I could feel physical sensations of dread shaking through my body like dirty grey wash water clogging my very being.

I was always nervous and highly strung, described as hyperactive by my parents – I would run not walk, could be quite intense at times, then break into uncontrollable rages. If I was a kid in the 90s instead of the 70s I would most definitely have been on ADHD medication. At school I couldn't concentrate, I was easily bored, I was creative and musical but struggled to mix and fit into the cliques of a small country school. One day I would have friends, the next those same friends would isolate from me and gang up. I did not understand and spent most of my primary school days in sick bay crying. I can still feel the soaking wet, hole ridden tissue in my small hand. I believed I had no worth even back then and the adults in charge simply didn't seem to notice.

At home on the farm, a remote sheep, wheat and cattle property, I lived with my parents, maternal grandparents and little sister. My dad eventually had a diagnosis of bipolar, but back then, undiagnosed, he calmed his demons with disappearances to the pub in town. We would sit in fear of when he would come home in an alcoholic rage, furniture broken and a sickening worry about the safety of my mum, a quiet beautiful soul. The next day us kids would know to stay away. I love my dad, we lost him this week, as I write this, to cancer. In his manic highs he could be terribly funny – he'd always make us kids laugh and do silly things and pull faces at us behind mum's back when she was trying to discipline us.

My grandmother had clinical depression and would take respite in the local mental health unit from time to time. Between my dad and grandmother, I was soon very familiar with the mental health unit, visiting one or the other, although they were never in there at the same time. Having a loved one with mental health issues taught my sister and I an innate sense and understanding of the intensity of moods, although this was quite anxiety provoking. One would have to sit in readiness, waiting to read dad's mood and rapidly assess what we needed to do to survive it. I always felt compassion for both of them. I knew who they really were as people rather than their ailment, but I did not have a full understanding until I was thrown into the pit of experiencing it myself.

Taking the St John's Wort, I thought ok, I can do this, I still seem to be ok, but slowly, slowly, I would find myself getting irrationally irritated at the tv, yelling abuse at the ridiculous ads. I became very cynical and angry, angry at the government, angry at the media, angry at society. "Have you taken your meds this morning Sharon?" "Yes", I lied.

Walking my kids to the school bus (from the outside I looked completely 'normal') sounds started to become louder, I could hear the tyres of vehicles on the road, the car's engine bellowed and reverberated through my body and I could not stand it. I could hear the leaves rustling in the trees, my footsteps on the gravel, I was hypersensitive to everything. People talking… about me? Racing heart, body shaking from the inside… constantly… I felt like I was removed from myself, a ghost, my spirit like a shattered mirror. Physical symptoms accompanied this despair I was feeling, I would rub my legs constantly, bite the skin of my lips, my hair started to fall out. I could barely talk, I could barely feed my family a meal, every little step through life was an effort. I was irritable with the kids but racked with guilt about this. I would apologise for everything. I would apologise for being their mother. I truly believed everyone would be better off without me.

The days turned into weeks then the weeks turned into months. I tried to brave it out, I didn't want to eat anymore, everything was bland, I wasn't interested, I wanted the pain to stop, I didn't want to be like this, no amount of Cognitive Behavioural Therapy (CBT) or mindfulness or deep breathing or fucking lavender oil could break into my hell. I could not shower, the effort was intense, washing my hair seemed like running a marathon. Dressing up, putting on jewellery and make up to go out seemed an impossible task. I could only manage a cup of tea and a biscuit at my husband's prompting. It was a despairing pain, a deep drowning engulfing black deathly hole of murky torturous pain, tormenting me all throughout my waking hours. There was no reason, my reasons for living had faded as the depths of despair took over my very being. I just could not face life, I decided my family were better off without me, even though a part of my brain was observing what was going on, I felt like I was split in two, there was me watching me. I was shattered… my mind was broken, but I was still there as an observer watching it unfold.

One day I could take no more, there was no reprieve, every waking hour was filled with despair and nothing was helping. In a teary daze, I took a vac hose, placed it in my car and left before my husband could get out of bed to stop me. I drove to a clifftop, maybe I could drive off? I drove towards the forest where I could run the car and go to sleep. I thought of the pain, I thought of the pain I would leave my children in – my mind was telling me it would be all right, they were better off without me, they would be ok… BUT I still had an inkling of the rational sparking through the darkness, and I drove to the emergency department at the hospital. I chose life. I accept I need meds and that's ok and I am still here.

Sharon Lomnicki is an Artist, Musician, Mum and Farm Owner. She is a dedicated Peer Worker currently working in Suicide Prevention and previously in the Housing and Accommodation Support Initiative. Sharon studied Art at University achieving a B.A. and DipEd. In her spare time she likes play drums with her rock band and ride her Harley Davidson. Sharon also has diagnosis of mental illness, and is passionate about dispelling stigma associated around mental health issues.

BACK FROM THE DARK SIDE
for Donna…
Glenn Cotter

It's dark, and there's no noise.
There's nothing.
What's happening, where am I?

I wonder if I'm dead.
No, can't be dead, still have thoughts… can't be dead.

I feel like I'm just floating somewhere, suspended in an incredibly thick black void. The darkness is so thick it's almost physical, surrounding me, I have no sensation of up or down or even of my own body.

It's so dark, what could have happened to me, does anyone know what's happening to me, can anyone hear me?

Time no longer means anything, nothing actually means anything, all I know is something must have happened, but what, and where am I?

A voice!! Very faint, where is it coming from, can't see anyone, can't see anything, but I can just make out a voice, soft, reassuring, comforting.

It's Donna's voice, I can't understand what she's trying to say to me but I know it's her, she's here with me, somewhere, telling me that everything's alright.

Then she's gone.

An eternity goes by, nothing but the thick black void of nothingness, my mind desperately trying to make some sort of sense of this but struggling to understand anything.

Wait, I hear her voice again, this time a little clearer, it seems to be all around me yet from nowhere specific.

"It's ok, you've had a motorcycle accident, you're in Hospital in ICU, but you're ok."

Why can't I see you, why can't I talk to you, what's happening to me?

Then the darkness embraces me again, this time though it feels slightly more comforting because now I know I'm alive at least.

Time seems to stand still, it's amazing where you mind goes when there is nothing for it to recognise or connect to. Okay, so I've had a motorcycle accident, where, what happened, shit, hope the bike is not damaged.

Your voice again, stronger this time, still can't make out what she is saying, but I can feel her nearby, her presence comforting, then the electric jolt as I feel her touch me, emotions overflow as I feel her touch, then she's gone again.

Don't go, please don't go, what is going on, why can I still not see anything, feel my body, understand any of this.

How badly am I hurt, can I still walk, will I ever be able to see again, the fear and confusion building, tormenting my mind, someone tell me something.

Slowly there's a sensation of moving, almost like being taken down from a shelf and put on a table… voices, telling me that they are going to do something, not sure what, can't really understand.

Then I feel it, someone is slowly wrapping their arms around me, rolling me, a soft voice in my ear, a man's voice, strong, compassionate, reassuring me that I'm safe. Then I hear another voice asking me to try to move my hands and feet, all the while the safe strong arms hold me.

Why can't I answer them, I try to talk but there is nothing, all I can do is nod weakly, then the arms are gone and I am slowly packed up and placed back onto the shelf until next time.

This goes on for what feels like a lifetime, and yet no time at all. Time has absolutely no relevance or meaning, it could be hours, days or weeks, I don't know.

More voices, your voice and wait, there's another one, that sounds like our son, Shaun, but it's so faint, distant, I can just hear you but I know you're there, I can hear you, I'm still here!

But where is here?

In time, the dark feels less oppressive, I can almost feel my own sense of being. Slowly the voices followed by the physical contact grow more frequent, the female voices clinical yet caring, the male voices always comforting followed by the gentle strength in their embrace.

I still have no idea what is actually going on, what are my injuries, what is my future, what happened to my bike, will I ever be able to ride again …

yes the brain takes you down some wild and wonderful rabbit holes, this must be how Alice was feeling at times.

Through it all your voice is the constant that drags me back from the wherever the hell I am. I can hear you, I can feel your presence, you are the constant in this nightmare.

More voices, they are taking me down from the shelf again to do something, not sure what, but there is someone who seems a little upset about something, a female voice full of authority asking questions… why doesn't someone ask me what I think? Oh yeah, I can't talk, that's right.

Time slips by, I find myself able to hear your footsteps approaching me, her presence lifts me from my darkness, sometimes there are other voices with her, I think I recognise some of them, but always her voice is strong and clear, something I can cling to, hold onto.

There are times that I feel lost, slowly drifting away to somewhere far away, but then I sense your footsteps followed by your presence and your voice pulling me back to where I am loved and needed.

Slowly I become more aware of the clinical voices and procedures, understand some of the questions, can nod my head or move my hands and legs in response to tasks and questions, all the while feeling safe in those strong anonymous arms, the caring yet powerful voice over my shoulder and in my ear, constantly assuring me that it's all good, I'm going to be ok.

Then the clinical voice in my ear…
"We are going to try to wake you up now, we are going to shine a light in

front of you, try to look at the light, focus on the light".

What light, what do you mean, what if I can't see the light? Fear and confusion set in, then slowly there it is a faint blur of light, slowly getting clearer, brighter, until it's almost blinding. I start to blink, trying to make it go away, but it is getting clearer, then there is a shadow beside it. What's that, is that a face, who are you, I don't know you, but wait a minute, I know that voice.

As the face becomes clearer I can almost feel my own body, looking up into the most beautiful face I have ever seen, then a voice saying… "Welcome back, we're so glad you could join us".

Seconds feel like hours as I try to get a grip of just what has happened, then the emotions just explode, and I am crying like a baby in the arms of the angel that I now know as the Head Sister in High Dependency Intensive Care Unit, the same angel who was there right through my journey.

But still confusion, why can't I speak, what are all these tubes and things, and oh my god, what is this pain!!!

Slowly and patiently she explains to me what has happened.

The 'darkness' was the result of a motorcycle accident, complications with injuries resulting in 3 separate cardiac arrests, before being stabilised, airlifted to Canberra and placed in an induced coma for 8 days. Injuries included 8 smashed ribs, bruised sternum, punctured lung and a torn trachea. Surgery to perform a tracheotomy was carried out during the week, explaining the inability to talk.

Throughout this ordeal you have been there at my bedside, you have been told by Specialists that they hold no expectations of my recovery. Your unbreakable bond and love through all this kept me here, of that I have no doubt.

My recovery stunned those who doubted, but you never did.

You have told me that in those darkest hours you accepted what could happen, asking only that if I couldn't come back 100%, that it was alright to not come back at all...

Over the next 3 years I experienced highs and massive lows; battling anxiety, depression and PTSD, and through it all you have been right beside me, even when I was so lost, I felt you there.

Every day I battle my demons, but I can now, because I know that you are there with me silently pushing me forward, your love and belief in me greater than anything I have for myself.

"Thank you," seems so inadequate.

You complete me, I am nothing without you.

Married to Donna for 32 years, daughter Sarah, son Shaun & granddaughters Madison, Jasmin, Tabitha & Ivy. Lives in Candelo on the NSW Far South Coast with Donna & five cats, I enjoy combining my love of motorcycles with my role as Community Ambassador with RUOK? & working as a Lived Experience Mental Health Peer Worker in the area of Suicide Prevention & Youth Work.

Making Sensory
Sandy Watson

Since childhood, I have experienced intense and prolonged struggles with mental distress. I struggled with intense fear, difficulties with my mood, visions and unusual beliefs, until I reached my fifties by which time the severity of my distress had significantly decreased, due to my persistent efforts in finding my own ways to ameliorate my distress.

I was on Disability Support Pension in my early thirties, having accumulated multiple psychiatric diagnoses, and taking medications ranging from barely tolerable to downright intolerable. I smoked heavily and used drugs and alcohol to get through the day. I felt hopeless about my future, surrounded by systemic messages of chronicity, severity, complexity, disability. I was unemployed and had been homeless on occasions. I was confused; I believed I was very ill and would never recover … I spent most of my days in bed, so impacted by my distress that it would take hours just to get up. The impacts on my life were devastating.

In my late thirties I chose to enter a drug and alcohol rehabilitation facility. Within a six-month period, I gave up cigarettes, drugs and alcohol: I could see that my life was getting worse; I needed to change if my life was to be about more than worrying whether there was food in the fridge.

After a difficult journey giving up drugs and alcohol, I wished I could also stop taking psychiatric medication. My mental distress was extreme (and supposedly chronic), I thought I would be on medication for the rest of my life. I knew that if I came off medications, I would definitely have to keep this from clinicians. It would be my secret mission. I wanted a better life; a life free from medication-induced migraines, fatigue, restlessness, dizziness, insomnia, drowsiness, dry mouth, low-blood pressure, high-blood pressure. I found it difficult to tolerate psychiatric medications, even in low doses.

After starting another medication that I experienced as disagreeable, I stopped taking it without consulting. I decided enough was enough. I marked the date that the new script was due for renewal on my calendar, so I would remember to ask my doctor for a repeat in five months' time. Over the next few months he thought I was doing well on this medication and I agreed! He said I was looking better. I told him I was tolerating it well!

When the time came, I threw the repeat script in the bin. There were no blood tests, so I kept up this ruse and he never knew that I wasn't taking the medication. I am not anti-medication, it has its place, but it wasn't working for me and there was no point with the pretence that it was. There was also no point discussing coming off medications at that time because the mental health system was so addicted to a bio-pharmaceutical mentality that I would have risked adverse consequences and exposing myself to suggestions I was lacking 'insight' as proof I was unwell and lacking capacity to make medical decisions in my own interests.

I started to figure out my own ways to deal with my distress. I didn't know how to do this, I had no role models: all of my 'mad' friends at the time were on medications, and they weren't talking about coming off.

I redesigned my life in many ways, pushing through my distress and gradually things got better. Without being hampered by unwanted medication effects, I could do more and try new things out. If something had a negative impact on my wellbeing, I didn't keep on tolerating it. I made many decisions: get regular sleep, have good friends, do things I enjoy. I let go of friends and social situations that weren't in my interests. I had more energy, I socialised more. I made new friends. I started to work for a few hours a week as an advocate. When I could comfortably work a few hours a week, I decided to go for harder jobs, eventually working up to six days a week in demanding advocacy roles with a lot of responsibility. I still experienced many challenges with my distress, with fears, unpleasant visions, depression, but I kept experimenting with different ways of responding to distress and pushing through, medication free.

The one thing that I worried about the most, in coming off medications, was what would happen if I became manic? I thought of all the things that had happened in my life when I was high, the damage to relationships and friendships, the homelessness, the financial costs, the hospitalisations, the things I said and did that were totally out of character and were embarrassing. I didn't know whether I would experience mania again, as most of the time it was caused by taking anti-depressants. Without taking anti-depressants, I was unsure whether mania was going to be a continuing issue.

I formulated a plan in the event that I got elevated again. If it happened, I was to go straight home and shut myself inside, no matter what, and then figure out what to do next. I always knew when mania was coming on – I had what I called 'manic-drift' -when aromas changed, colours were brighter, sounds were louder and I was feeling wonderful, on top of the world.

One night I was out with friends to watch the Mardi Gras parade when I noticed my 'manic-drift' coming on. I went home before the parade started. When I got inside, it felt intense. Mania came on in a matter of a few hours, out of nowhere. I decided to sit on my bed and stay there, not leave home, and not do anything stimulating. In that moment, I realised that for me, this wasn't any different to managing migraines, which I had dealt with since I was eleven.

When I have a migraine, I do anything to shut down stimuli; lights out, blinds drawn, no sound, no movement, and I lie still in a quiet place. I am used to doing this. I suddenly understood that my 'manic-drift' could be interrupted by restricting sensory stimuli, the same thing I do with migraines. An over stimulation of sensory stimuli could be responded to with the same strategy as managing a migraine by shutting down the stimuli.

With this new realisation in mind, I sat on my bed for three days, and confidently did nothing! No T.V. No radio. No reading. No drawing. No telephone calls. No going out for a walk or spending time in my favourite café. I was determined to starve myself of sensory stimuli – there's no fire without kindling for the flame. I had years of practice behind me with migraines, often spending days in bed so it wasn't that hard to do (except it was boring!).

Three days after this started, it stopped. I succeeded in shutting down the manic-drift. This was the first time I managed this experience without medication. In the past I would be swept up in the elevated state, staying up all night, quickly ploughing through my money, painting at the same time as reading a dictionary whilst trying to solve the worlds' problems, perhaps ending up in hospital.

Today I don't see this experience as a 'mood disorder', but rather an intensification of sensory stimuli. I know what to do if it comes on. It has taken discipline and patience to address this issue, but I already had the skills and knowledge that I acquired with migraines.

Looking back over my madness life, I am grateful that I had the courage to stop listening to others' perspectives on my distress, to the multiple diagnoses and prognostications, to the term 'chronic' and all that was packaged with it, to take my own counsel in relation to my distress, to listen to my body as to what I need to do in any given situation.

Last year I competed in an international dragon boating regatta in Florence, on the Arno River, with a team I love. I spent days doing street photography in Rome and Florence and had a fantastic time with two wonderful friends visiting ancient sites like Pompeii, the Colosseum, and touring Tuscany.

P.S. A note to my struggling self, thirty years ago: Thank you for your courage, even when you had no idea that it could get better. Thanks for not giving up, even when your life was difficult, and you couldn't see the point in going on. Thanks for making sense of your distress in your own distinctive ways, for trusting in your own judgement about what to do and how to live. Thanks for striking your own path. Whilst there are difficult struggles today, they are less intense, less frequent, and are easier to respond to and resolve.

Sandy Watson is a Co-Director of inside out & associates australia. She has lived with extreme states of distress since childhood, and has found her own ways of dealing with her distress. Sandy identifies as being a trauma survivor and is in recovery. She is a lived experience educator, facilitator, and course writer, living in Sydney.

Acknowledgements

This book would not have been possible without a bunch of people who provided support, advice and encouragement behind the scenes.

Firstly, we would like to acknowledge Tyler Wagner and Authors Unite for the inspiration and information which was the impetus for making this book happen.

Much appreciation also to Natalia Jerzmanowska, Col Jennings and Tim Heffernan for their assistance and advice regarding editing and other project-related decisions.

A big thank you to Mahlie Jewell for bringing imagination, honesty and patience to the process of creating the cover and typesetting the contents.

And finally, our heartfelt gratitude to the 307 people who backed Our Own Words on Kickstarter, many of whom are listed below. (Some people chose not to be named in this book.)

Ailsa

Ashleigh Allan

Sue Allan

Thu and Chris Andersen

Julie Anderson

Kate Andrews

Lisa Archibald

Liz Asser

Aunty

Cassie B

Matt Ball

Michelle Banham

Frank Barnes

Karlen Barr

Niki Barr

Lisa Baston

Joel Beeson

Rhondda A. Bell

Brett Bellingham

Brendan Bennett

Sharon Bent

Berry Family

Lizzie Blue

Susan Bonar & Jennifer Coote

Nicole "Nikki" Bond

BPD Awareness ACT

Liz Boston

Kylie Boucher

Glenda Michelle Browne

Fiona Browning

Kristie Bull

Clare Burford

Emma Cadogan

Dr Catherine Camden Pratt, AThR

Elise Cannon

Chelsea Cappetta

Caretakers Cottage

Deb Carlon

Sarah Carter

Liam Casey

Kyla Cassells

Charise

Bianca Childs

Marie Choi (Maz)

Pamela Coburn

Michelle Cole

Wendy Cooper

Andie Coughlan

Isabelle D.

Michael A Daley

jo davies

Alastair Deards

Maryanne Doherty

Carolina Dowling

Lorna Downes

Rosemary Durbidge

Marion Drake

Leonie Dunn

Katie Edwards

Mag Eli

Nat Ellis

Priscilla Ennals

Cindy Eugene RN

Kimmy Ellyse Eveland

Michelle Everett

Simone Firmin-Sarra

Carolyn and Frank Fuller

Tricia-Leanne Gehrig

Zoe Glen-Norman

Luca Schilling Gonçalves

Sandra Goode

Gotherella

Ben Gourley

Dr Penelope Goward

The Graham-Bish Family

Grand Pacific Health

Flick Grey

Mia Gyaneshwar

Suzi H.

Lesley Halliday

Julz Hatherly

Tim Heffernan

Mary Henry

Petra Chloe Hill

Janelle Hint

Tyneal Hodges

Annette Hope

Lisa Howell

Bronwyn Howlett

Suze Hutchison

Elizabeth Huxley

Annaleisa Ienco

Carolyn Ienna

Kim Irwin

Fay Jackson

Janice

Jess

Natalia Jerzmanowska

Mahlie Jewell

Vicki Johnson

Jay Jolliffe

Zach Jones

Melanie Jorgensen #LapsforLachy

Jennie K

Dr Leonie Katekar

Dr Claire Kelly

Kellie Kembrey

Ally Kernagham

Rose L.

Tara Laing

Duncan Large

Lou Larkin

Tina Lathouras

Leanne

Karen Leask

Amy Leigh

Ione Lewis

Ella Linwood

Philippa Lohmeyer-Collins

Georgia Lonergan

Leanne Lonergan

Larissa MacFarlane

Lyn Mahboub

Laura Maher

Marcie

Mandy Marsters

Leah Martin

Andrea McCloughen

Alison McInerney

Fiona Mckay

Leah McKenner

Sarah McKenzie

Julie Millard

Joanne Millington

Evie Milonaki

Stephanie Mitchell

Dr Ros Montague &

Peter Bazzana

Jodi Morriss

Thayna Natal

Nathe

Nateve

Carol Nemes

Kerrie Noonan

Kim O'Malley

One Door Mental Health

Sophie Peacock

PeerZone

Carmen Perrin

Jenelle Pike

Daryn Poulden

Hayley Purdon

Celine Quinn

Karl Bruce Raams

Reeces-Peaces

Anna Richards

Rachel Rive

Robert

Daneka Rose

Anne Samuelson

Justin Scanlan

Shahaf Ben Shalom

Paul Shearer

Rosa Simon

Kellie Simpson

Jenny Smith

Jennie Somerville

Jo Sommer

SA Lived Experience Leadership
and Advocacy Network (LELAN)

Jenny Stathopoulos

Sam Brhaspati Stott

Wei-May Su

Xia Li Summerfield

Lindy Sutherland

Dr Mark Tayar

Celia Taylor

Victoria Tipton

Anastasia Tjhin

Michelle Townsend

Trevanis – CEO Hypermania
Enterprises Ltd

Emma Tseris

Emma Tucceri

Jenny Valdivia

Peter Valpiani

Joanne Veltkamp

Karen Walcott

John Wand

Natalie Watson

Sandy Watson

Sue Watson

Wesley Mission

Mark R Wilder MSW-RSW

Rosie Williams

Johnny Windus

Gini Witt

Cheryl Wittingslow

Carol Woolley

Diane Wendy Wright

Donna Wright

Marianne Wyder

Beate Zanner

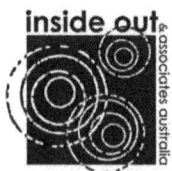

www.insideoutconversations.com.au

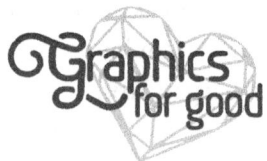

www.graphicsforgood.com.au